# THE USE AND ABUSE
# OF
# SPORT AND PHYSICAL ACTIVITY

**Earle F. Zeigler,**
**Ph.D., LL.D., D.Sc., FNAK**
**The University of Western Ontario**
**London, Ontario, Canada**

**TRAFFORD**
2011

Order this book online at www.trafford.com
or email orders@trafford.com

Most Trafford titles are also available at major online book retailers.

Printed in the United States of America.

ISBN: 978-1-4269-7300-0 (sc)
ISBN: 978-1-4269-7301-7 (e)

Trafford rev. 10/12/2011

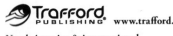 www.trafford.com

North America & international
toll-free: 1 888 232 4444 (USA & Canada)
phone: 250 383 6864 ♦ fax: 812 355 4082

## Dedication

In a world facing an uncertain future, a field historically known as physical education faces an uncertain future as well…

I dedicate this book to all those who have contributed over the years to help *physical activity education* (including educational and recreational sport) to serve humankind in the best ways possible

# Table of Contents
# (and Conceptual Index)

# Preface

Titling this book *The Use and Abuse of Sport and Physical Activity* was not the original title I chose. I had decided to call it *Values or Disvalues in Human Physical Activity*. However, I finally realized that I wanted more than a few sport philosophers and historians to read what I had to say on the subject. Even that prediction might have been optimistic…

Nevertheless, when one talks or writes about "the use and abuse of something," the underlying rationale soon reverts to whether that "something" has value or not to the person who chooses to use it or abuse it. In this case the purpose of this book is to discuss thoroughly how humankind has used physical activity throughout history–and how humankind has abused it in relationship to the subject of (developmental) physical activity.

Values are principles or standards of behavior that people consider to be important or beneficial. They are basic and are an integral part of every culture. A person is a member of a culture and typically holds beliefs and assumptions about it and the world in which it functions. People in such a culture typically share a common set of values and these values form the basis for their behavior. If this were not so, a particular culture would disintegrate because its members would not know what values they stood for in their lives.

Values are more general and abstract than norms. They explain what should be judged as good or evil. Norms are more general rules for behavior and devolve to rules in specific situations. Values that seem beneficial and important will be viewed positively. Conversely, undesirable values will be viewed negatively. *The latter might also be termed as "disvalues."*

In summary, the values they hold convey to people what is good and what is important in their lives. If something is useful, for example, they value it. If something is desirable, they value it. Speaking personally, if an observer knows my values, he has a good idea as to how I will act in specific circumstances. Speaking personally, if a value seems good to me. I will treasure it.

Developmental physical activity (e.g., work, exercise, sport) have had a long history on Earth. They have been of greater or lesser importance to people over the millennia. Sport, for example, from a very humble beginning where cave men or women played a competitive game, has somehow developed to the point where a man can make many millions of dollars just by throwing an inflated pigskin through the air. Or he could be a millionaire many times over–if talented enough!–

by persistently keeping a hard-rubber disk from sliding through his legs on ice into a rectangular net that he is "protecting." However, to this day he must be a male member of the species to earn such a large amount of typically greenish paper known as "currency of the realm" to the cognoscenti.

To earn such large amounts of money, you usually have to do or accomplish something very important in our complex society. Nevertheless, how could such seemingly simple maneuvers with—say—an object of one type or another be worth so much to the performer? The answer is simple or complex depending upon how or where it is done—and under what circumstances. This is the interesting, perhaps ridiculous, aspect of the development of a game or sport generally that has grown so disproportionately important during the 20$^{th}$ century of humankind's life on a speck in the universe known as Earth. Parenthetically, Earth is located in an infinite galaxy of astral bodies known colloquially as the universe. Or is it multi-verse?

To bring my narrative "back to Earth," I will now "begin at the beginning" by telling you just how I decided to try to affirm this evident truth (first to me!) and now to you, the reader. I thought the world (Earth!) would be in better shape by the time I died (ha!), but it actually appears to be in a "worse mess" than when I started in my profession 70 years ago. Disturbingly, also, the news of "fresh disasters" is arriving faster and with greater detail because of improved communication globally. And such news is increasingly more of "a mess" daily no matter how or from what direction you look at it! Natural disasters simply occur, but the "impending disaster" I am fearing has been brought about by a creature known as "man" or "woman" (mostly man!).

O.K. So let us assume that impending disaster looms. What about it? And where do sport and related physical activity (exercise!) as **valuable** physical activities fit into this discussion? Since the evolution of our species on land began, human physical activity in sport, exercise, and physical recreation has become an increasingly important and vital aspect of the life of those "humans" who are now in "essential control" of the planet.

My chosen task in this book is to show that sport and related physical activity assumed greater or lesser importance starting with primitive societies and continued in later societies on down to the present day. (I am now recommending the term "developmental physical activity" as a disciplinary name for the field.) Physical activity is literally a social force impacting society generally, and also as a vital concern for those desiring to employ it professionally in a variety of ways within society. Such activity has been used by people of all ages in a variety of ways as the human species evolved and these creatures lived out their lives.

However, as is the case with so many facets of life on Earth, such involvement can be used beneficially or misused to the subsequent improvement or detriment of humankind. It is my thesis that we are using it well in some ways, *but that we are also abusing it badly in others!* In the case of competitive sport, I believe we have gradually abused it (i.e., perhaps reaching a stage where could well be doing more harm than good with it). Conversely, in the case of related physical activity (i.e., regular exercise or "physical activity education") in the developed world, I believe humans are too often "abusing it by first not understanding it and then by not using it more intelligently"! (Ironically, in the "undeveloped world," people often get *too much* "exercise" just to stay alive!)

As I see it, with sport we are using it, or people are "using us", but not to its best advantage. They are not getting the most value from it. They may even be getting negative effects or disvalue from it. In the case of exercise, in the so-called advanced societies, we are using it insufficiently--and therefore not to its best advantage either. How this has happened since earliest times is the task I have chosen for myself to explain in this book.

Please understand this, however: I don't for a moment argue here that (1) the proper use of sporting activities throughout the earth's affairs could be a panacea for all of the world's ills, the elixir that would create a heretofore unknown era of good will and peace worldwide. I do believe, however, that wisely employed it could enrich lives "healthwise" and recreationally for many more millions than it is doing presently.  In addition, I do assert (2) that *the wise use of exercise and sound health practices throughout people's entire lives would indubitably go a long way toward keeping people happier and healthier in lives extended in years because of this type of life practice.*

What I am arguing is that, employed properly and correctly, sport and related physical activity–*as one of a number of vital social forces (e.g., nationalism, ecology)*– could contribute to the improvement of the current situation enormously. Moreover, I believe that the active use of competitive sport worldwide to promote what have been called *moral* values, traits or attributes, as opposed to so-called *socio-instrumental* values, would create a social force of such strength and power that humankind might be helped as it confronts the social and physical devastation looming ahead. At the very least, I believe such active promotion would delay to a considerable degree the onset of what promises to be a destructive societal situation.)

15

Such an "untenable societal scenario" has been described vividly by Walter Truett Anderson in the essay "Futures of the Self," taken from *The Future of the Self: Inventing the Postmodern Person* (1997). He sketched four different scenarios as postulations for the future of earthlings in this ongoing adventure of civilization. Anderson's "One World, Many Universes" version is the most likely to occur. This is a scenario characterized by high economic growth, steadily increasing technological progress, and globalization combined with high psychological development. Such psychological maturity, he predicts, will be possible for a certain segment of the world's population because "active life spans will be gradually lengthened through various advances in health maintenance and medicine" (pp. 251-253)

Nevertheless, a problem has developed with this dream of individual achievement of inalienable rights and privileges. In a world where globalization and economic "progress" seemingly must be rejected because of catastrophic environmental concerns or "demands," the Captain Kirk, bold-future image could well "be replaced by a post-modern self; de–centered, multidimensional, and changeable" (p. 50).

The systemic-change force mentioned above that is shaping the future, this all-powerful force may well exceed the Earth's ability to cope. As gratifying as such factors as "globalization along with economic growth" and "psychological development" may seem to the folks in a coming "One-World, Many Universes" scenario, there is a flip side to this prognosis. Anderson identifies this image as "The Dysfunctional Family" scenario. All of these benefits of so-called progress are highly expensive and available now only to relatively few of the six billion plus people on earth. Anderson foresees this as "a world of modern people happily doing their thing; of modern people still obsessed with progress, economic gain, and organizational bigness; and of postmodern people being trampled and getting angry" [italics added] (p. 51). As people get angrier, present-day terrorism in North America could seem like child's play.

Hence, the charge I have given myself is to make the case that civilization is steadily giving evidence that (1) the social phenomenon known as competitive sport is largely being used incorrectly, and (2) the social phenomenon known as developmental physical activity (and related health education) is being employed insufficiently and inadequately. Both of these activities promoted one way or another through physical activity education and related health instruction could combine to provide much greater value to humankind. They could be a social force that used properly could go a long way to the creation of a better, more peaceful world. *Presently I believe that the relationship between these two aspects (i.e., sport and exercise) of a potentially most powerful social force is "out of joint" in the developed world. It must be rectified for the ultimate good of humankind!*

Exactly how to tackle this enormous problem (i.e., bring the "two aspects of this powerful social force" back "in joint") is the tremendously complex task that faces a world that doesn't appear to recognize the depth and severity of the problem. First, it would be necessary to "enlighten" a substantive majority of the world's population, and then the actual "enlightenment" would have to result in the implementation of these two "practices" to a desirable extent in people's daily lives. Hence it appears that my task is to first try to explain how "*it*" happened (i.e., this "disjointedness"). Then, when I have delineated the problematic situation as clearly as possible, I will try to explain exactly what would have to happen so that the two aspects of this powerful social force can be balanced in a way that will *contribute to* humankind survive–and not continue to *hinder*–in the years ahead.

Succinctly, then, I will seek to seek to trace the problem historically. I will describe the social forces that affect society, and I will explain how the social force of **values** influences all other values. As I get to the 20th century, I will explain why America, despite its' professed good intentions and actions–and often executed ones!–shares a good portion of the blame for humankind's dilemma in the developed world.

> Note: Because I divided my professional career equally between America and Canada, and also because the situations are similar, much of this material applies to the Canadian scene as well. In addition, a number of references made apply to Canada.

Next I will single out sport and physical activity education–as social forces based on developmental physical activity–portraying how they (together!) have increased in influence down to the present day. In the process I will explain how completed research is telling us that sport is being used ever more to promote what have been designated as "socio-instrumental" values rather than to promote so-called "moral" value development. (Note: The terminology here is a bit confusing as it seeks to convey specified meanings.)

Next to last, I will try to explain precisely what changes would have to occur in sport to convince people as to the direction we **must** take. Then I will describe what type of physical activity education seems necessary and most desirable for the very large majority of people who are either "under-exercised" or "over-exercised" (in each case because of their imposed or elected lifestyle).

Admittedly, all of this sounds like an impossible task. To me, however, it does seem possible–even plausible!–if we work collectively to promote the appropriate level of physical activity for people of all ages throughout the world.

You may ask how this could be possible if the social force of *values* is so dominant thereby influencing all other social forces "beneath" it on the prevailing scale of values. The answer is that values are *not–should not be!–*rigid and inflexible in all regards. They should be human-made! As we understand what works for the "desired good" in our daily lives for the betterment of humankind, these values should be implemented!

Hence, if people can be convinced to promote the "right kind" of competitive sport and developmental physical activity (exercise!), this type of "adjustment" could conceivably bring about a desirable amount of specific value improvement and ultimate *overall* change in the world's prevailing value structure.

I conclude by asking: "What have we to lose, if we don't do everything possible to bring these two related aspects of a growing social force into an acceptable alignment?" I can only conclude that–unless we tackle this issue positively and definitively–*we may lose everything*!"

Earle F. Zeigler
2011

# Prologue

## A Brief History of "PE"
## (Which Is Basically "TNEMEVOM")*

Blank, sometimes designated as _____, but who really should be called **tnemevom** (which is quite difficult to pronounce), has had both a glorious and a shameful existence historically. IT (tnemevom) is a part of the very nature of the universe. This is an incontrovertible fact. IT is involved with both the animate and inanimate aspects of the cosmos. IT is a basic part of the fundamental pattern of living of every creature of any type that has ever lived on Earth. Early men and women knew IT was important, but IT was often not appreciated until IT was gone, or almost gone. Civilized men and women used IT extensively in the early societies, as did the Greeks and Romans and all others in the East. Some used IT vigorously, but others used IT carefully and methodically. IT was used gracefully by some, ecstatically by others, rigorously by many when the need was urgent--and regularly by most who wanted to get the job done. IT was called many things in various tongues. But, strangely enough, IT was never fully understood.

The time came when IT was considered less important in life, although people still admired IT when used skillfully on special occasions. Some seemed to understand IT instinctively, while others had great difficulty in employing IT well. IT was eventually degraded to such an extent that well-educated people often did not think that IT had an important place in preparation for life. Others gave lip service to the need for IT, but then they would not give IT its due. Others appreciated its worth, but felt that IT was less important than many aspects of education. But IT persisted despite the onset of an technological age. Some called IT calisthenics. Others called IT physical training. A determined Germanic group called IT gymnastics. A few called IT physical culture, but they unfortunately were thought to be men of "ill repute." Others felt that IT had been neglected in the preparation of the human for life. So, they did IT a "favor" and called it **PHYSICAL EDUCATION**!

### The Aftermath of a New Name.

Physical education (formerly known here as IT) gradually prospered to a degree with this name, although it was embarrassing because it did classify **PE** as a second class citizen. This idea persisted even though, early in the 20th century, the field was called "a physical education" which was "justified." This canceled out *forever* out the belief that the mind and body were separate. However, as they say, long–held beliefs die hard! Nevertheless, physical education struggled on… Then an unexpected development happened. As a result of a modicum of prosperity, physical education "spawned" offshoots. Two of these offshoots had been closely related to **PE** for a long time; they were known as dance and athletics. These were two new offshoots. One became known as recreation, and the other as health & safety education. Our hero (physical education, or **PE**!) helped to develop them quite a bit, and they--in their gratitude--helped physical education too as they themselves developed.

Then, after two great and numerous lesser wars, and the impact of other social forces on society, physical education--still a second-class citizen among educators--discovered that its offshoots (recreation and health & safety education) had grown quite large and important in the world. They too were anxious to become first-class citizens, and they made loud noises on occasion to inform all that they deserved priority in life. Many people--at least a goodly portion of them-- recognized that they were right. But times change slowly, and the education of human creatures was only slowly be influenced by this recognition.

During this same period of time, two other phenomena occurred that held great import for physical education. PE's brothers & sisters, athletics and dance, had been performing so well that they had steadily grown strong and powerful. Athletics (or **"SPORT"** as it is called on continents other than North America) looked at PE and said "What a dull clod art thou!" What athletics (sport) meant was that physical education, or blank, or _____ (tnemevom) (which is quite difficult to pronounce) wasn't very exciting. Actually it could be quite dull with its repetitive exercises and endurance activities that promote muscular strength, flexibility, and cardiovascular efficiency. Sadly enough, **DANCE** (his other relative) seemed to feel the same way. PE realized, of course, that s/he had a responsibility to teach young people about tnemevom in schools, but could understood it was so much more thrilling to perform for the cognoscenti (as dance), and even for the multitudes (as sport). So dance said: "I'm an art. So I think I'd be better served by joining my fellows in one of the performing arts centers springing up around me." Even athletics (sport) "moved in" on many PE classes…

If matters weren't bad enough, Sputnik went up in the late 1950s--and the world has not been the same since. "Science" became the watchword in the 1960s and has continued as such ever since. Professional preparation for physical education was criticized sharply in a report by a Harvard president. The result was that never-too-important **PE** (**tnemevom** or blank) soon discovered that many university professors no longer wanted to be known as "physical educators." They felt a bit ashamed to be called "that"! They thought it hurt their chances for status and much-desired grant funding. So the name "kinesiology" was proposed by some like-minded, "badgered Texans under siege" by state legislators attacking the shallowness of courses that included the word "education" in them. "Kinesiology" was thus to be a panacea for beleaguered academics ("if they don't know what it is, how can they criticize it?").

This "study of movement" name, the word taken from the Greek language, had been *the name of a course* in the professional physical education curriculum for a century. It could be "fathomed" quite well kinematically, but not by 99% of us kinetically. Now it was also to become **THE** name for the department or school in a university. What they were saying was, "Let PE be for the schools; kinesiology should be the "in name" for us scientists in the universities! (Question: What then about the social-science and humanities aspects of our field?) Still another faction seized upon the term "kinetics" and the word "human" before it. This sounds good too, but it is identical with both the prevailing name for dynamics with physics and that for studying rates of reaction within the field of chemistry. (Question: Why should we muddy the waters further?)

Still further, in addition to the effort to "scientize" "good old PE" that started in the "sixties," a solid thrust in the 1960s designed to promote solid *theory* to practice in the realm of physical education and athletics administration got caught up and slowed down by both "scientification" and budgetary restrictions in the 1970s. When this movement returned in the 1980s, somehow the emphasis was soon much greater on commercialized sport than physical education and athletics in educational institutions.

## The Unhappy Plight of Physical Education (good old "PE").

All of this made physical education (**PE**) or blank, or _____, or **tnemevom** felt very sad. In fact, PE became more worried than ever before. **PE** could look back at a long heritage since the beginning of the universe and just *feel* important. However, **PE** could rationalize that people simply misjudged the importance of tnenevom whose motives were pure. People always seemed to treat him as stupid, even though they knew that they needed such involvement. Also, when seemingly intelligent people discussed **PE,** their lips tended to curl even though they might themselves be fat (or obese) or even diabetic. Thinking about the proverbial rose, **PE** wondered if he would "smell as badly" with another name. Maybe another name was needed, even a new disciplinary name such as "phyactology" (Fraleigh). Such a name made sense, even though "savants" laughed when it was first proposed…

**Time for Reflection**.

And then PE began to think deeply--that is, as deeply as a second-class citizen can think. **PE**'s male component, had a "twin sister". This female creature often made different noises as she went her own way. She had been telling him, "the male **PE**", that he couldn't see the forest for the trees. "**PE**," she said, "we have really been fools, and we merit our plight. We have been so stupid that we haven't been able to spell out what we really should have been called--**tnemevom**--it is, to to be sure, but we have had it completely backwards.

Crestfallen, but with a rising sense of elation, tnemevom came to life all at once. S/he took a deep breath, tensed muscles, and executed a back somersault with a half twist. S/he assumed new dignity almost immediately, as s/he realized that here was a new name that was quite simple to pronounce. It was ***MOVEMENT***! From that day forward, s/he vowed to carry out the field's true function more purposely than ever before. S/he recognized that s/he could still relate effectively to brothers, sisters, and "offshoots." But, more importantly, s/he realized that there was more to "movement" than push-ups and jogging, as truly important as these parts of movement might be. S/he realized that s/he had physiological aspects, anatomical aspects, psychological aspects, philosophical aspects, sociological aspects, historical aspects--and many more than could be counted on the fingers of two hands.

This was a most important realization for ***MOVEMENT*** (formerly spelled tnemevom), but he didn't rush off blindly to proclaims his glory to the world. S/he had learned a good lesson. This time it would be under girded by a sound scientific and scholarly basis. This time the field's name would be spelled correctly and the case for recognition would be soundly based. The field could be defined as "the interaction of the human and his/her movements" (Paddick, 1967). Or, if you will, broaden Kenyon's (1968) term to "human movement arts and sciences."

Good old "**PE**" suddenly felt very tired. Should s/he change names again? "Kinesiology" sounded too complicated and esoteric. What we are fundamentally, s/he thought, is human physical activity in sport, dance, play, and exercise. Our knowledge base comes from what might be called the movement arts and sciences, a field that can help humans throughout their entire lives.

S/he realizes that those would do good in this world cannot expect others to roll stones away from their path. It's a hard road that lies ahead. Perhaps I'm not up to the challenge, s/he thought… But if this road is to be traversed, it must be done by a determined, united group of qualified, professional physical activity educators. These stalwarts will be engaged in ***Physical Activity Education*** or ***Movement Education***.

Let's not debate the issue any longer, s/he decides, since the sun is already quite high in the sky… Long live ***tnemevom*, because without *IT* you're dead!**

EFZ
2011

# Chapter 1
# What Are Humans?

A book about something called "use and abuse of" or "values and disvalues" in human physical activity such as exercise and sport may not be destined to make even the bottom rung of the bestseller list. Yet, oddly enough, if such a book were well-written and sufficiently informative, it should challenge the #1 spot. I write this because most of us know that the world is in "big trouble", *and yet practically no one is looking in this direction for possible answers.*

The interesting thing is that people should be looking in this direction for two pieces of advice. The first is that people in the "advanced" world must follow a wise pattern of "developmental physical activity" if they wish to long, healthy, and satisfying lives. The second piece of advice is that people are neglecting the first piece of advice just mentioned and are turning instead to dubious types of involvement or "non-involvement" with innumerable competitive sports. Nevertheless it is not that sport is bad in itself–far from it. It's simply that sport is being "abused" or "maltreated" as people only watch it or use it incorrectly.

A logical progression on this subject would be to have an opening chapter that first asks the question: "What Is the Universe"? In other words, I should start from the very beginning! However, I didn't major in astronomy at my university. Even if I had done so, I probably would have had difficulty describing the universe to a generally educated reader. Frankly, I couldn't answer this question satisfactorily myself! So, I turned to Google on the Internet and simply typed "The Universe" in the line with the clicking cursor. As a result I discovered reams of information.

Now, if convenient, I urge you to do just that–right now! Unless I am mistaken, you will find two videos available to you in response. They are on either the first or second page that comes up. Click on the left one, the longer one that lasts about 10 minutes while playing good music. When I did this for the first time, I was completely overwhelmed by the unbelievable enormity of it all. All that I can say is: "Wow"! So, if you have a computer sleeping nearby, please do this. Then I truly think you will be more ready to start reading Part 1 below…

To continue: It would be a good bet that the large majority of people on Earth don't give much, if any, thought to the question "What Are Humans?" raised by the title of Part 1 above on the preceding page. We *are* humans: we *are* at the top of the food chain–and that's it! And yet *your* answer–and a *collective* answer to it–are absolutely vital and fundamental to our future on this very tiny planet in an unbelievably vast "multiverse". Living our lives from day to day we sometimes forget that the planet Earth originated more than 4 billion years ago--or maybe even earlier!.

Early man and woman, we are told, had their beginnings some one million years ago and have used crude tools for less than half that time. Three hundred thousand years have elapsed since the mutation of sub-man into man. We now know that many tribes roamed and then settled at various points in prehistoric Europe during a warming trend at the time of the Wurm Glaciation of the late Pleistocene Epoch from 35,000 to 25,000 years before the present.

## The "Adventure of Civilization"

The adventure of civilization began to make some headway because of now-identifiable forms of early striving which embodied elements of great creativity (e.g., the invention of the wheel, the harnessing of fire). The subsequent development in technology, very slowly but steadily, offered humans some surplus of material goods over and above that needed for daily living. Nevertheless, the beginnings of the first civilizations as we know them are actually less than 10,000 years ago. (See, for example, *Bahn, 2000.*)

For example, the early harnessing of nature created the irrigation systems of Sumeria and Egypt, and these accomplishments led to the establishment of the first cities. Here material surpluses were collected, managed, and sometimes squandered; nevertheless, necessary early accounting methods were created that were subsequently expanded in a way that introduced writing to the human scene. As we now know, the development of this form of communication in time helped humans expand their self-consciousness and to evolve gradually and steadily in all aspects of culture. For better or worse, however, the end result of this social and material progress has created a mixed agenda characterized by good and evil down to the present. The prevailing religions are the product of the past 2,500 or so years. As types of political state go, democracy is the youngest of infants, its official origins dating back only several centuries to the late 18th century. Is it any wonder that perfection appears to be a long way off?

On this subject Muller concluded that "the adventure of civilization is necessarily inclusive" (1952, p. 53). By that he meant that evil will probably always be with humankind to some degree, but it is civilization that sets the standards and then works to eradicate at least the worst forms of such evil. Racial prejudice, for example, must be overcome. For better or worse, there are now more than six billion people on earth, and that number appears to be growing faster than the national debt! These earth creatures are black-, yellow-, brown-, red-, and white-skinned, but fundamentally we now know from genetic research that there is an "overwhelming oneness" in all humankind that we dare not forget (Huxley, 1967).

## The Ways Humans Have Acquired Knowledge

Royce (1964) stated that there are notably four basic means whereby people sought to surmount the obstacles preventing them from acquiring fact, knowledge, and wisdom about the universe, about Earth within it, and about people and other creatures residing on this planet:

> (1) thinking, that has become known as rationalism
> (2) intuiting or feeling, that is designated as intuitionism
> (3) sensing, that means of knowing called empiricism
> (4) believing, that tendency of humans to accept as truth that which is stated by a variety of presumably knowledgeable people--an approach known as authoritarianism

## Four "Historical Revolutions" in the Development of the World's Communication Capability

As we move along with our consideration of the ongoing change that has taken place throughout history, the developments in communication are such that we humans can only marvel at the present status of opportunity for human growth that has been created. Isaac Asimov has delineated these stages as follows:

> (1) the invention of speech,
> (2) writing,
> (3) mechanical reproduction of the printed word, and now

(4) to relay stations in space creating a
    blanketing communications network that
    is making possible a type of international
    personal relationship hitherto undreamed
    of by men and women (Asimov, 1970).

Humans we, who tend to think we are "the greatest," may be excused from wondering occasionally why the "Creator" took such a laborious route with many odd variations of flora and fauna to get to this point of "present greatness." For hundreds of thousands of years, the forebears of present-day humans chipped flints to their tools. However, as they used their brains and their hands, both an enormous biological advantage, it is now evident that in their primitive self-consciousness they were not living only for the moment like their contemporaries, the apes.

As various world evils are overcome or at least held in check, scientific and accompanying technological development will be called upon increasingly to meet the demands of the exploding population. Gainful work and a reasonable amount of leisure will be required for further development. Unfortunately, the necessary leisure required for the many aspects of a broad, societal culture to develop fully, as well as for an individual to grow and develop similarly within it, has come slowly. The average person in the world is far from acquiring full realization of such benefits. Why "the good life" for all has been seemingly so slow in arriving is not an easy question to answer. Of course, we might argue that times do change slowly, and that the possibility of increased leisure has really come quite rapidly once humans began to achieve some control of their environment.

Of course, there have been so many wars throughout history, and there has been very little if any let-up in this regard down to the present. Sadly, nothing is so devastating to a country's economy. Also, in retrospect, in the Middle Ages of the Western world the power of the Church had to be weakened to permit the separation of church and state. This development, coupled with the rising humanism of the Renaissance in the latter stages of that era, was basic to the rise of a middle class. Finally, the beginnings of the natural sciences had to be consolidated into real gains before advancing technology could lead the West into the Industrial Revolution (Toffler's "Second Wave").

Admittedly, permitting a conscious choice between alternatives goes as far as permitting the presence of "population pockets" where there is a demand to give creationism co-equal status with the teaching of a Darwinian long-range approach to human evolution in the schools. As humans we, who tend to think we are "the greatest," may be excused from wondering occasionally why the "Creator" took such a long and laborious route with so many odd variations of flora and fauna to get to this point of "present greatness." The power that these advantages provided humans was steadily combined with technological advancement, but somehow only offered minimal levels of freedom. As mentioned above, the early development of language as a means of communication was vitally important. This distanced sub–humans even more from the apes as cultural evolution became much faster than biological evolution. In a sense, culture brought with it "good news" and "bad news." The bad news was that humans are now to a large degree trapped in a world that they themselves created. Fixed habits and beliefs are strong inhibitors of change, growth, and what might be called progress.

The good news is that, very slowly, change did occur; growth did take place; and to most people such change and growth represented true progress. For example, prehistoric humans did interbreed, and in this way broadened their genetic base. In the final analysis this lends credence to the present-day argument introduced above that humans today--brown or yellow, black, and white--are indeed one race. This fact helps us to appreciate the development of worldwide cultural evolution. Unfortunately, however, progress has never been a straight-line affair. In the final analysis, this must be the answer for those of us who idealistically thought that the world would be in quite good shape by the year 2000! It may also provide some solace to those of us who wonder why education finds it so difficult to get sufficient funding; why professors in so many countries must often assume a "Rodney Dangerfield complex". Little wonder that physical activity education, including educational sport, despite consistently mounting evidence of the "worthwhileness" of developmental physical activity--so often finds itself in dire straits within the domain of education and in the eyes of the public.

World society is obviously in a precarious state. It is therefore important to view present social conditions globally. Throughout this volume I will be emphasizing that competitive sport has developed to a point where it has worldwide impact, and also human physical activity should be so organized and administered that it truly makes a contribution to what Glasser (1972) identified as "Civilized Identify Society"–a state in which the concerns of humans will again focus on such concepts as 'self-identity,' 'self-expression,' and 'cooperation.'

Postulating that humankind has gone through three stages of society already (i.e., primitive survival society, primitive identity society, and civilized survival society in which certain societies created conflict by taking essential resources from neighbors, Glasser theorized that the world should strive to move as rapidly as possible into a role-dominated society so that life as it is presently known can continue "wholesomely" on Earth.

## Historical Images of Humans' Basic Nature

Any effort to delineate the present status of Western man and woman must include also some consideration of the postulations that have been offered concerning the basic nature of a human. In the mid-1950s, Van Cleve Morris presented a fivefold, chronological series of overlapping philosophical definitions including analyses as (1) a rational animal, (2) a spiritual being, (3) a receptacle of knowledge, (4) a mind that can be trained by usage and that functions within a body, and (5) a problem-solving organism (1956, pp. 22-22, 30-31). Within such a sequential pattern, the task of the physical activity educator/coach might be to help this problem-solving organism to move efficiently and with purpose in exercise, sport, and expressive movement. Of course, such experience would necessarily occur within the context of the individual's socialization in evolving world society.

A bit later, Berelson and Steiner (1964) traced six images of man and woman throughout recorded history, but more from the standpoint of behavioral science than Morris' philosophically oriented definitions. These images were:

(1) The philosophical image (the equivalent of Morris' "rational animal"). In Classical Greece, ancient man and woman distinguished virtue through reason.

(2) The Christian image (Morris' "spiritual being") which contained the concept of "original sin" and the possibility of redemption through the transfiguring love of God for those who controlled their sinful impulses.

(3) The third image appearing in sequential order on the world scene during the Renaissance was the political image (a behavioral orientation in contrast to Morris' "receptacle of knowledge" a philosophical categorization) through which humans, through power and will, managed to take

greater control of the social environment. In the process, sufficient energy was liberated to bring about numerous political changes, the end result being the creation of embryonic national ideals that co-existed with earlier religious ideals.

(4) The economic image of the human (contrasted this with Morris' "mind that can be trained by usage") emerged during the 18th and 19th centuries, one that provided an underlying rationale for economic development in keeping with the possession of property and material goods along with improved monetary standards.

(5) The psychoanalytic image emerged in the early 20th century. Berelson and Steiner postulated the stage that was not included in Morris' classification. It introduced another form of love—that of self. Instinctual impulses were being delineated more carefully than ever before. The result was that people were led to believe that childhood experiences and other non-conscious controls often ruled people's actions because of the frequently incomplete gratification of basic human drives related to libido and sex.

(6) Finally, because of the rapid development of the behavioral sciences, they postulated the behavioral-science image of men and women (roughly the equivalent of Morris' "problem-solving organism," but with an added social dimension). This view of the human characterized him or her as a creature continuously adapting reality to his or her own ends. In this way the individual is seeking to make reality more pleasant and congenial and-to the greatest possible extent--his own or her

own reality (Berelson & Steiner, 1964, pp. 662667).

## The Seven Rival Theories About Human Nature

Keeping Berelson and Steiner's six images of human nature listed above in mind, in trying to answer this question about human nature more precisely, I eventually decided to include further the insightful work of Leslie Stevenson. He suggested that there are seven rival theories that postulate an answer to this basic question about the basic or intrinsic nature of man (generically speaking) (1987). Each of these prognostications is saying in essence: This is "the hand that we've been dealt," and "this is how we can best react to it what it is telling us":

1. Plato: The Rule of the Wise
2. Christianity: God's Salvation
3. Marx: Communistic Revolution
4. Freud: Psychoanalysis
5. Sartre: Atheistic Existentialism
6. Skinner: The Conditioning of Behavior
7. Lorenz: Innate Aggression

As I continued, it seems that my purpose here will be best served as well by a brief consideration of each of the seven theories delineated by Stevenson about (1) the nature of the universe, (2) the nature of men, (3) a diagnosis of the situation humans face, and (4) a prescription of what each "prognosticator" thought should be done to bring about the best result.

*Theory #1: Plato–The Rule of the Wise.* Following the above sequence, Plato, for example, is arguing that that (1) this is my theory about the universe we live in (i.e., his theory of another world of "existing Forms"), (2) our nature as humans as being dualistic (i.e., mind and body), (3) the belief that these Forms are ideals about the parallel world, and (4) the prescription that the only way the world is going to "make it" is if the wisest of men rule it. (Note: I suppose in a way that's what we are doing in a democracy where we elect a person as head of state for a period of time…)

*Theory #2: Christianity–God's Salvation.* Moving ahead to theory #2, Stevenson stated next that Christianity also had a theory about (1) the nature of the universe, (2) what humans were like in this environment, (3) how God has explained what is wrong with man and women, and (4) what he/she needs to do about it to be saved. It does seem that there are so many differences and subdivisions by people subscribing to this theory that it is difficult to spell out the "essentials." God created the universe that is "up there" somewhere in space and in time. This universe is identified with God, a deity that is both transcendent and immanent.

The nature of man is explained as a creature made in the image of God and who is destined to have control of the rest of God's creation. However, in a seeming contradiction, he/she is also "continuous with it." True Christians believe there is life after death through a process of resurrection. A crucial point in Christianity's view of human nature is that the human is free and has the ability to love while finding true purpose (i.e., love of God).

Proceeding to the "diagnosis stage" of this theory, we find that the human has from the beginning misused his God-given right of free will by initially making the wrong choice. In this way he has sinned and the relationship with the Creator was upset. Hence, nothing he/she does will bring about "perfection" in life and living. The human alienated himself from God by assertion of the will.

What is the prescription then? Humans must look to God for ultimate salvation. The New Testament of The Bible helps humanity to find a way to eternal salvation by explaining that God sent his son, Jesus, to earth to restore the disturbed relationship that developed through suffering and atonement for the evil of man. Each person on earth must individually accept "God's redemption" provided to him/her by the life and resurrection of Jesus. In this way a way of life has been provided for the true believer.

*Theory #3: Marx–Communist Revolution.* It is interesting to note that Karl Marx was born a Jew in a German family that converted to Christianity. Eventually devoting himself to the philosophy of Hegel, Marx believed that humankind was destined to go through certain stages of development, each possessing a "character" of its own. This was in essence a pantheistic belief asserting that God was the whole of reality. However, when Hegel's followers split into two camps, Marx followed the thought of Feuerbach that led to the belief that religion was really identified with alienation from earthly affairs. Hence, he opted for a more radical position that it was up to humans to help move the development of humankind to a new stage of development that envisioned social progress yo be tied to material rather than spiritual progress. This resulted in the ongoing application of a materialistic interpretation of history that led to the rise of the interpretation of history as being too materialistic thereby leading to the idea that capitalism must be eliminated as the prevailing economic theory.

Marx claimed that his theory of the universe explained historical development scientifically; thus, he searched for universal laws underlying social development. An "Asiatic phase" gave way to an ancient era that eventually merged with a feudal period. Then a socialistic phase set in to be followed inevitably by a capitalistic one as worldwide commerce gradually developed. Ultimately, as we know, capitalism was to be forced to give way to communism. There were laws of history operating here, he claimed, arguing that this study of history was truly a science that could be tested by evidence. His theory appears to overemphasize the materialist conception of history asserting that material life's mode of production is what gives society its "character" socially, politically, and "spiritually.

Although capitalism has its problems, it is still in an extremely strong position in the world with some of the avowed communistic countries adopting many of its practices. However, this struggle is far from over as the gap between rich and poor accentuates with the middle class being squeezed increasingly between them in so-called developed countries. Thus, it could be argued that a type of socialism will be needed to satisfy "the multitudes in their search for a good life."

In the theory of man that is postulated with Marxism, the future is deterministic as man progresses through various stages of history being exhorted to help the process along. Some urge that the change be brought about precipitously, whereas others seem willing to let history evolve. The essentially social nature of the human is viewed as fundamental. We learn through our relationships with others. In addition, different from all other creatures, we have learned to produce a good deal of what is needed for our subsistence. Human development could be considered a social development brought about by men and women possessing a strong sense of social activism. The study of sociology is obviously extremely important.

Marx's diagnosis of the human's plight is that he/she (Western human actually) has become alienated within world society because of the gradual adoption of capitalism as the economic system to emulate. It is difficult to understand exactly how such alienation from one's self and Nature has occurred. However, we can assume that this alienation might be from what humanity has created, and this alienation is also from the basic nature of humans. It may be possible to get some help by looking to the main points of the Communist Manifesto. Difficulty arises, however, when we conjecture that Marx's concern would be nicely rectified by turning everything over to the State instead of leaving so much in the hands of private enterprise. However, we can understand that Marx was "loudly" decrying the abuses displayed in the early stage of capitalism when men served *only* as an economic end.

Moving from diagnosis to prescription with Theory #3 about human nature is a simple matter. An economic system where capitalism prevails is a bad development, and it must eliminated while something better is introduced. That "something" is to be "the Communist Revolution"! The debate really warms up at this point. Social democracy is too "gentle" and "long-winded" to bring about the necessary change; so, "bring on the Revolution"! The aftermath of this overthrow would be a social system in which humans would be "regenerated" and function in a society where ideally and eventually the State as supreme power would fade away. Considered in the light of day, we cannot but agree that the envisioned end is indeed glorious. However, considering the nature of the human, we must be suspicious of this demand to "throw out the baby with the bathwater and begin all over again." Nevertheless we know that a large segment of the world's population is living in societies that claims to have done just that…

*Theory #4: Freud–Psychoanalysis.* Sigmund Freud and his theory of psychoanalysis are important to us in this discussion because through his work he made such an enormous contribution to people's understanding of themselves as they live in an evolving world. Freud was a scientist who evidently didn't spend much time on metaphysical speculation about the nature of the universe, He was purported to be an atheist who viewed the world as a phenomenon in which such sub-phenomena are governed by what are called physics and chemistry. Humans evolved on this planet and are presumably subject to any laws that prevail.

The subject becomes much more complicated, however, when we shift our attention to humans. Stevenson decided to subsume Freud's ideas about humans under four categories: (1) application of the principle of determinism, (2) the postulation of unconscious mental states arising from the first category, (3) his theory of the instincts human instincts or "drives," and (4) his developmental theory of individual human character.

Determinism meant that every "mental event" was a result of something previous that occurred in the human mind. The second category delved into mental states by asserting that "the mind is not co-extensive with what is conscious or can become conscious." There are dynamic, unconscious aspects of the mind that can influence action. This does not mean, however, that a Platonic dualistic theory (mind/body) of the human is true; the principles of physiology still hold sway. He postulated, however, that the mind has three major structural systems: (the *id*, the *ego*, and the *super-ego*. The drives of the id need immediate satisfaction; the ego has to do with the human's relationship to the outside world and thereby has a direct influence on any possible anti-social drives, for example, of the id. The superego, as he postulates is that part of the ego that mediates between the outside world and the person's id. It seems confusing, but the task of the superego is to supervise the ego by projecting society's moral rules and norms to help the id "restrain itself" as the human faces society daily. Simple, n'est-ce pas?

As if this weren't enough for one man's theoretical contribution. Freud also opined about the great importance of instincts or "drives" as motivating forces within the human mind. The one that has received the most attention perhaps overemphasis, of course has to do with the human's sexual drive.

We can't leave our all-too-brief discussion of Freud's work without inclusion of Freud's developmental theory of the individual having to do with human character. He theorized about the respective influences of experience and heredity as the child and youth goes through the several stages of development on the way to maturity. It is obvious that Freud presented humanity with much to ponder over on the subject of human nature.

Moving to the "diagnosis stage" with this summary of Freud's contribution, it is immediately obvious that the well-adjusted person would exhibit a harmonious relationship among the various "parts" of the brain (as postulated by Freud) as the individual confronts "the outside world." A person can talk about it glibly using the terms supplied, we know that "making it all work" to the individual's and society's best interest is another matter. For example, there is the concept of "repression" that might be used as a defense mechanism when the person is under stress and can't seem to adjust to society's demands. However, as we mature, we must learn to cope with the conditions that confront us to "maintain control" within our familial and external environments. To what extent society "may have gone wrong" is another matter.

To undertake some "prescribing" after brief diagnosis, Freud would have us maintain a harmonious state between the several "parts" of the mind. In addition, there needs to be reasonable harmony between the person and the world. Freud did not get into the question of possible social reform, but devoted a large portion of his time and effort to the psychoanalysis of patients. Further discussion of this treatment would serve no purpose in this volume devoted to human values and disvalues related to sport and physical activity.

*Theory #5: Sartre–Existentialism.* Philosophers identified with what has been called existentialism are a "very mixed breed." However, there does appear to be consensus that this approach is concerned with the individual, the purpose of his/her life, and the amount of freedom granted to said person. Interestingly there are both Christian and atheistic existentialists!

Jean Paul Sartre's "brand" of existentialism denied the existence of a God, and he inquired as to what that "non-existence" meant for the individual human. Most importantly this theory of a God-free universe meant that there are no such things as "objective values" that control human life. Thus, if life has no purpose, Sartre described it as "absurd." For him this meant, therefore, that the individual is free to choose his/her life values.

How, therefore, do we describe the nature of this creature that has evolved and whom we call "man"? We are here. But there doesn't seem to be any reason for our presence. This means that, since we are sentient. if we are to have a purpose we had best get at its creation. Right now we really don't know what we ought to be! However, it does seem apparent that we have been "condemned to be free." So what are we going to do about it?

The result seems to be that the human been challenged with responsibility because of the freedom somehow granted to him or her. It's sort of a "don't just sit there; move it!" situation. Hence, what we do, or don't do, assumes great importance to ourselves–and to others who may be in our path as we wander through life.

The diagnosis of the plight that has befallen man is crucial. We can deceive ourselves and say we are not free, but that would be stupid. Sartre calls such deception "bad faith," but admits that many people end up trapped in their life situations in this way.

Unfortunately, however, the rejection of the bad-faith approach does not offer the human a clear and definitive assessment of the self. Defining the self is truly elusive, because, as Stevenson (p. 97) asserts: "human reality is not *necessarily* what it is, but must be *able* to be what it is not." This seems to boil down to a case of "striving mightily" to be truly free and in the process to avoid "bad faith."

Okay… Where does this leave us when we come to the question of prescription for the individual subscribing to the existentialistic stance in life? The situation is that there are no basic values so far as we can see. So we have to figure what life amounts to all by ourselves. As an individual, therefore, I should try to avoid "bad faith" and do my level best to be "authentic" in whatever I choose to do with my life. This is the challenge handed over to us if we accept this philosophical stance. So be it!

*Theory #6: Skinner–The Conditioning of Behavior.* To this point the efforts included have been those of men approaching the question of human nature philosophically to a large degree. The next one included here takes a somewhat more scientific tack into what has become the discipline of psychology. Here we will condense very briefly the efforts of B. F. Skinner, an experimental psychologist, studies that led him to make generalizations about human nature from the area known as "the behaviorist tradition."

Skinner was preceded in his endeavors by J. B. Watson and others who sought to carry out their research empirically as "the study of consciousness." However, Skinner in a 1913 paper stated that they\se scholars had reached the point where they could not agree on methodology in their research. Hence, he argued that it was time to "go outwards" and study human *behavior*. It could be observed and analyzed better than the assessment of previous introspective analyses. In addition, the importance of environment in human development, as over against heredity, was singled out by Skinner. This question is still open, however, in the 21st century.

With regard to *the theory of* the universe underlying Skinner/s approach, his endeavor was simply an affirmation of thought stating that scientific method must be used to determine what nature, including human nature is all about. The search must be for uniformities and general laws that apply under all circumstances. In this way theory grows and expands as the human seeks to control the environment and thereby thrive on into the indeterminate future. At present people make value judgments and then seek to induce others to accept their stated position on "this and that" about the world. If some practice works efficiently. And effectively (beneficently) in society, that means it should be evaluated as "good." To summarize, Skinner as a scientist was searching for uniformities among phenomena looking to understanding, relating, and ultimately controlling the world.

Insofar as Skinner's study of human nature went, he viewed the individual as literally

"unexplainable". Keeping genetic factors in mind, he looked for environmental causation of human behavior. He believed (1) that there were scientific laws to be determined that governed human behavior, and (2) that these laws explain the relationship between these environmental factors and subsequent human behavior. In assessing these statements, we are somehow left, however, with the possibility that analysis of behavior doesn't "explain it all"–that there may also be "innate factors" that come into play as well.

Reflecting on a *diagnosis* of Skinner's theory, we are confronted with the clash between his thought and that of Sartre. Skinner believes in the determinism "of it al," and Sartre tell us that we are "condemned to be free"! Are humans "free agents" or not? What a difficult question to answer! And yet we  might as well "throw in the towel" if we concur with Skinner in this regard. On the other hand, however, the "loneliness" of the person in the world postulated by Sartre is "scary" as well. Whether an intermediate position is possible appears to be the question. If there was a "social cause" for my "dubious action," why can't I be held at least partially responsible by society?

Now let us consider the *prescription* stage in regard to Skinner's deterministic position at hand. The human is faced with a world that "determines" where he/she is heading. Much of this looks very worrisome indeed. Do we "give in to it," or do we work mightily to create a situation where we find longevity and "life satisfaction" as the world evolves? Skinner would have us improve the present situation by conditioning people's behavior in a variety of ways (i.e., inducements, "positive" propaganda). This all sounds most encouraging. However, there is just "one hitch"! Someone, or some group of people, would have to "call the shot," so to speak. This is indeed a tricky situation in which to be placed. I, as author, find myself of two mind as to my decision. Finally, I must opt for "the dignity of freedom to choose myself"!

Theory #7: Lorenz–Innate Aggression. Finally in this "you pay your money; you take your choice approach" I am offering here, we come to the work of Konrad Lorenz, a man who called himself an ethologist and argued that the happenings of early childhood are basic to a person's subsequent philosophical and later scientific development. This attempt to study the character of animals scientifically by describing what happens when the environmental situation of creatures changes or is altered.

The assumption was that the instinctual behavior patterns of a particular species occurred as a result of the individual's genes evolving down through the ages. Hence it is easy to understand why Darwin's *Origin of Species* (1859) caused such a furor when the human's evolution through so-called natural selection was propounded. I won't attempt to repeat the four empirical propositions tested by this assertion. Suffice it to say that "the world" has not been the same since this contradiction of Christian doctrine,

As the work of Lorenz proceeded, he concentrated on the aggressive behavior of humans and what this meant for "the human condition." Hence as this biological scientist considered the nature of the universe, he found that creatures of this Earth had developed hereditary movements that were instinctive and innate even though many of these human creatures' drives gave the appearance of spontaneity. The four most importanr drives of feeding, reproduction, flight, and aggression combined to provide a sort of unity to human nature.

Here Lorenz's special study of human aggression is being considered–a major instinctive drive. He examined how various species had learned to "protect their territory" in order to survive down through the ages. The "necessary" aggression had its bad points and its good points, as Lorenz saw it, but overall under "controlled circumstances" such aggression may be desirable when not overly destructive.

Moving along to Lorenz's theory of human nature, it is obvious that it correlates strongly to behavior patterns exhibited by other animals. Nature's causal laws work on us too, and we deny this similarity to out individual and collective peril. This doesn't mean, however, that some people have not developed a high degree of personal control in regard to their aggressive nature. A highly interesting theory emerges from his deliberations and studies, however. Somehow we appear to have developed an almost innate drive leading to aggression toward our own species–perhaps even more so than is the case with many other animals! This came about possibly when other tribes threatened a specific tribe, and over the millennia the "warrior instinct" emerged as basic to survival. Certain types of "communal defense" may have preordained people to aggression for survival purposes.

The diagnosis of this development postulated by Lorenz may mean that literally weak human insofar as possessing deadly appendages were concerned had no need to worry especially about "human internecine warfare" before the "age of deadly weapons" appeared to present humankind with the possibility of complete annihilation and self-destruction. Hence, we seem to have ended up with a good reason for humans to follow the advice of Dr. Hawking that earthlings shouldn't ne in too big a hurry to relate to species on other planets!)

Proceeding to what might be a possible prescription for the human being who conceivably might have acquired through the passage of eons an innate aggressiveness toward his *"foreign"* neighbor in a circumscribed world where "neighbors" are within easy striking distance, what can be recommended? Might it be possible somehow to eliminate this frightening aggression? We can't build impregnable walls, nor can we drugs that will pacify us. If one culture were to try to "breed aggression out" of its population, who's to say that other groupings would reciprocate? It seems that only more self-knowledge resulting from research might help people understand their feelings and motivations better. In this way we might promote significant good will leading to international peace.

Interestingly, and hopefully, there were groups of British and American scientists, lead by M. F. Ashley Montagu and others who argued conversely against the man-is-bad view of humankind. They argue that the question is still debatable, far from having been decided convincingly that the future looks bleak for the human species. Undoubtedly the twentieth century has been a bleak one, and the beginning of the twenty-first one hasn't seen many positive signs yet of a new, more peaceful age. However, we must proceed on the basis that "there is hope yet" for a more peaceful world in the future.

## Two Basic Historical Questions

To this point we know that we are organisms, living creatures, who have reached a stage of development where we "know that something has happened, is continuing to happen, and will evidently continue to happen." However, underlying my entire analysis I am searching for the answers to *two historical questions*: First, did humans in earlier times, equipped with their coalescing genes and evolving **memes**, enjoy to any significant degree what discerning people today might define as "quality living?"

> (Note: Memes are sets of "cultural instructions" passed on from one
> generation to the next; see below, also.)

Second, did earlier humans have an opportunity for freely chosen, beneficial physical activity in sport, exercise, play, and dance of sufficient quality and quantity to contribute to the quality of life (as viewed possible by selected sport philosophers today)?

(Note: Of course, the phrasing of these questions--whether humans in earlier societies enjoyed quality living, including fine types of developmental physical activity--is no doubt presumptuous. It reminds one of the comedian whose stock question in response to his foil who challenged the truth of the zany experiences his friend typically reported: "Vas you dere, Sharlie?")

What makes a question about the quality of life in earlier times doubly difficult, of course, is whether present-day humans can be both judge and jury in such a debate. On what basis can we decide, for example, whether any social progress has indeed been made such that would permit resolution of such a concept as "quality living" including a modicum of "ideal sport competition" or "purposeful physical activity and related health education."?

There has been progression, of course, but how can we assume that change is indeed progress? It may be acceptable as a human criterion of progress to say that we are coming closer to approximating the good and the solid accomplishments that we think humans should have achieved both including what might be termed "the finest type" of sport competition.

## The Difficulty of Defining Progress

Despite what has just been stated above the "forward leaps" that have been made in the area of communication, any study of history inevitably forces a person to conjecture about human progress. I first became truly interested in the concept of progress when I encountered the work of the world-famous paleontologist, George Gaylord Simpson (1949, pp. 240-262). After 25 years of research, he offered his assessment of the question whether evolution represented progress. His study convinced him that it was necessary to reject "the over-simple and metaphysical concept of a pervasive perfection principle." That there had been progression he would not deny, but he inquired whether this really was progress. The difficulty comes, he argued, when we assume that change is progress; we must ask ourselves if we can recommend a criterion by which progress may be judged.

We are warned that it may be shortsighted for us to be our own "judge and jury" in this connection. It may well be an acceptable human criterion of progress to say that we are coming closer to approximating what we think we ought to be

that it has a general validity in evolution." Thus, throughout the history of life there have been examples of progress and examples of retrogression, and progress is "certainly not a basic property of life common to all its manifestations." If it is a materialistic world, as Simpson would have us believe, a particular species can progress and regress. There is "a tendency for life to expand, to fill in all the space in the livable environments," but such expansion has not necessarily been constant, although it is true that human beings are now "the most rapidly growing organism in the world."

It is true also that we have made progress in adaptability and have developed our "ability to cope with a greater variety of environments." This is also progress considered from the human vantage point. The various evolutionary phenomena among the many species, however, do not show "a vital principle common to all forms of life," and "they are certainly inconsistent with the existence of a supernal perfecting principle." Thus, Simpson concludes, human progress is actually relative and not general, and "does not warrant choice of the line of man's ancestry as the central line of evolution as a whole." Yet it is safe to say that "man is among the highest products of evolution . . . and that man is, on the whole but not in every single respect, the pinnacle so far of evolutionary progress" on this Earth.

With the realization that evolution (of human and other organisms) is going on and will probably continue for millions of years, we can realize how futile it is to attempt to predict any outcome for the ceaseless change so evident in life and its environment. We can say that we must be extremely careful about the possible extinction of our species on Earth, because it is highly improbable, though not absolutely impossible, that our development would be repeated. Some other mammal might develop in a similar way, but this will not happen so long as we have control of our environment and do not encourage such development. Our task is to attempt to modify and perhaps to control the direction of our own evolution according to our highest goals. It may be possible through the agency of education, and the development of a moral sense throughout the world, to ensure the future of our species; one way to accomplish this would be to place a much greater emphasis on the social sciences and humanities while working for an ethically sound world-state at the same time.

### The "Tragic Sense of Life" (Muller)

One realizes immediately, also, that any assessment of the quality of life in prerecorded history, including the possible role of sport in that experience, must be a dubious evaluation at best. However, I was intrigued by the work of Herbert

Muller who has written so insightfully about the struggle for freedom in human history. I was impressed, also, by his belief that recorded history has displayed a "tragic sense" of life. Whereas the philosopher Hobbes (1588-1679) stated in his *De Homine* that very early humans existed in an anarchically individualistic state of nature in which life was "solitary, poor, nasty, brutish, and short," Muller (1961) argued in rebuttal that it "might have been poor and short enough, but that it was never solitary or simply brutish" (p. 6).

Accordingly, Muller's approach to history is "in the spirit of the great tragic poets, a spirit of reverence and or irony, and is based on the assumption that the tragic sense of life is not only the profoundest but the most pertinent for an understanding of both past and present" (1952, p. vii). The rationalization for his "tragic" view is simply that the drama of human history has truly been characterized by high tragedy in the Aristotelian sense. As he states, "All the mighty civilizations of the past have fallen, because of tragic flaws; as we are enthralled by any Golden Age we must always add that it did not last, it did not do" (p. vii).

This made me wonder whether the 20th century of the modern era might turn out to be the Golden Age of the United States. This may be true because so many misgivings are developing about former blind optimism concerning history's malleability and compatibility in keeping with American ideals. As Heilbroner (1960) explained in his 'future as history' concept, America's still-prevalent belief in a personal "deity of history" may be short-lived in the 21st century. Arguing that technological, political, and economic forces are "bringing about a closing of our historic future," he emphasized the need to search for a greatly improved "common denominator of values" (p. 178).

However, all of this could be an oversimplification, because even the concept of 'civilization' is literally a relative newcomer on the world scene. Recall that Arnold Toynbee (1947) came to a quite simple conclusion about human development is his monumental *A study of history*--that humankind must return to the one true God from whom it has gradually but steadily fallen away. An outdated concept, you might say, but there is a faint possibility that Toynbee may turn out to be right. However, we on this Earth dare not put all of our eggs in that one basket. We had best try to use our heads as intelligently and wisely as possible as we get on with striving to make the world as effective and efficient--and as replete with good, as opposed to evil, as we possibly can.

Here we might well be guided by the pact that Goethe's *Faust* made with the Devil. In this literary masterpiece from the pen of the German literary figure, Johann Wolfgang von Goethe (1748-1832), we recall the essence of the agreement struck by Faust with the then-presumed actual purveyor of the world's evil. If ever the time were to come when Faust was tempted to feel completely fulfilled and not bored by the power, wealth, and honor that the horned one had bestowed upon him, then the Devil would have won, and accordingly would have the right to take him away to a much warmer climate. Eventually, as the reader may recall, by conforming to the terms of the agreement, Faust is saved by the ministrations of the author. Yet, we at present can never forget for a moment that previous human civilizations were not miraculously saved! Literally, not one has made it! Thus, "Man errs, but strive he must," admonished Goethe, and we as world citizens today dare not forget that dictum.

# Chapter 2
## What Are the Values Held by Humans?

### Defensible Ethical Decisions
### Require Careful Thought
### and A Wise Choice of Values

Values are principles or standards of behavior that people consider to be important or beneficial. They are basic and are an integral part of every culture. A person is a member of a culture and typically holds beliefs and assumptions about it and the world in which it functions. People in a culture typically share a common set of values and these values form the basis for their behavior. If this were not so, a particular culture would disintegrate because its members would not know what values they stood for in their lives.

Values are more general and abstract than norms. They explain what should be judged as good or evil. Norms are more general rules for behavior and devolve to rules in specific situations. Values that seem beneficial and important will be viewed positively. Conversely, undesirable values will be viewed negatively. The latter might also be termed as "disvalues."

In summary, the values they hold convey to people what is good and what is important in their lives. If something is useful, for example, they value it. If something is desirable, they value it. Speaking personally, if an observer knows my values, he has a good idea as to how I will act in specific circumstances. If a value seems good to me. I will treasure it.

Humankind has won a recognizable semblance of victory over what is often a harsh physical environment despite the frequent tricks played on us by "Mother Nature." However, it is obvious that in society today that people have not yet been able to remove much of the social insecurity present in their lives as they seek to live together peacefully and constructively. Almost everywhere one may turn, there is evidence that a crisis in human values exists. Wholehearted agreement with this dictum– being handed down arbitrarily here from "on high that such a crisis exists--is not required at this point. Nevertheless, a good case can be made that the most persistent problem any person faces today is the necessity for a regular, ongoing determination (or reaffirmation) of his or her personal values. These *personal* values as they are designated here, constitute *all* of the "major" and "minor" values that individuals hold implicitly based on their background experience.

In an effort to help society, many philosophers and theologians have searched through the ages for an acceptable (normative) ethical system that espouses a moral base upon which people could and should base their conduct. However, as Earth move along in the 2000s of the Common Era (C.E.), there is still no non-controversial foundation on which the entire structure of ethics can be built. Perhaps there will never be...

In considering humankind's basic problems, a leading philosopher, E.A. Burtt, in his *In Search of Philosophical Understanding* (1965) believed that the greatest *danger* to our future "lies in the disturbing emotions and destructive passions that he [man, primarily] has not yet overcome; the greatest *promise* lies in his capacity for a sensitive understanding of himself and his human fellows." If indeed "distorting emotions and destructive passions" do represent the greatest danger to the future, the application of a sound ethical approach to personal and professional living could be of inestimable assistance to people who are truly seeking a "sensitive understanding" of themselves and their associates.

However, as life becomes ever more complex in the early 21st century, there are at least *eight* major ethical routes to decision-making extant in what we call the Western world (Graham, 2004). Everything considered, it can be argued reasonably that this "ethical smorgasbord" confronting humankind is highly confusing. Also, because the achievement of consensus has eluded humankind these thousands of years, problems of greater and lesser importance related to ethics and human values abound. These are all problems that should somehow be resolved through sound ethical decision-making.

Further, the present way in which a young person initially learns how to make rational ethical decisions in North American society must be described as inadequate. A child and young person typically presumably acquires such competency--or lack of it!--implicitly through everyday experiences, including what direct guidance his/her elders or contemporaries may offer. This laissez-faire approach is truly insufficient as the young person seeks to develop reasoning powers. Society is faced, therefore, with an ongoing situation where it should be helping young people to learn *explicitly* how to develop their own conscious convictions in which the mind *leads* and the emotions *follow* to the greatest possible extent. The next step here is to review briefly how society has tried to be of assistance up to the present time.

## Values: Objective or Subjective?

Now that we have an overview of the question "What Are Humans?", it is time to ask "What are these values held by humans?" Values are principles or standards of behavior that people consider to be important or beneficial. They are basic and are an integral part of every culture. A person is a member of a culture and typically holds beliefs and assumptions about it and the world in which it functions. People in a culture typically share a common set of values and these values form the basis for their behavior. If this were not so, a particular culture would disintegrate because its members would not know what values they stood for in their lives.

Values are more general and abstract than norms. They explain what should be judged as good or evil. Norms are more general rules for behavior and devolve to rules in specific situations. Values that seem beneficial and important will be viewed positively. Conversely, undesirable values will be viewed negatively. The latter might also be termed as "disvalues."

In summary, the values they hold convey to people what is good and what is important in their lives. If something is useful, for example, they value it. If something is desirable, they value it. Speaking personally, if an observer knows my values, he has a good idea as to how I will act in specific circumstances. If a value seems good to me. I will treasure it.

A question arises. In addition, are values objective or subjective–that is, do values exist whether a person is present to realize them or not? (This is not the same question as whether a falling tree in a forest makes a noise when no one is there to hear it!) Or is it people who ascribe value to the various relationships they have with others--and possibly also with their physical environment? If a human activity fulfills objectives (leading to long-range aims) inherently valuable to people, then it should be included in formal and informal education offerings throughout their lives--*perhaps whether people of all ages recognize this value or not. If, on the other hand, if it were somehow proved that such an activity in has little value, and that the majority of people sees no need for it, then according to the subjective theory of value, it should be eliminated.*

Another facet of the question of values refers to their qualitative aspects. An individual may desire certain things in life, whereas other things may be desirable mainly because society has indicated its approval of them. Actually, a continuous appraisal of values and norms occurs. (Keep in mind what sociology tells us about the difference between values and norms. Norms relate to values, but they also result in the establishment of laws. For example, in a democracy personal security is valued very highly. So the norm established is that the individual shall be protected from harm, and laws are created to see to it that such laws are upheld.)

If a value exists in and for itself, it is said to be an *intrinsic* value. One that serves as a means to an end, however, has become known as an *instrumental* or extrinsic value. When intense emotion and appreciation are involved, this gradation of values is called aesthetic. Physical activity education (including sport) offers many opportunities to realize aesthetic values, although many well-educated people--according to our society's *norms*--view the entire field of aesthetics far too narrowly and thereby confine such values to experiences in the fine arts and literature. Every culture seeks to develop its own hierarchy of values, and any profession's responsibility, for example, along with its related disciplines, is to discover through scholarly endeavor and research what it has to offer society. If its practitioners are able to truly prove its worth to people based on such sound scholarship, then those practitioners will also have to work to help in the development of people's affirmative attitudes toward the inclusion of what that profession stands for in people's life patterns.

Perhaps the least understood, yet most persistent problem that any professional faces, for example, is the necessity for the ongoing determination (or reaffirmation) of his or her personal (or individual) values. We all hold such values implicitly as part of our background experience. Eventually, as we become professionals in some field of endeavor, we should also explicitly determine our value orientation as a fundamental aspect of our relationship to the clients that we serve. In the case of the educator, this person should be fully cognizant of how such a decision possibly contributes to the achievement and possible inculcation of these values in the lives of students or people with he/she works.

This is not a simple matter to resolve. Ever since I became involved with this aspect of my profession, it soon became evident that people were confused and uncertain in this regard; they simply had not worked out a coherent, consistent, and reasonably logical approach to the values that they held in life. I knew that each one of us had a "built-in" set of values, but most people simply couldn't express what it was they were working toward in their lives. In most instances the values that they held had been achieved *implicitly* along the way, or perhaps they had simply been "handed" someone's or some organization's position, creed, or purpose. Only in rare instances had an opportunity been provided to think this subject through carefully and systematically so an *explicitly* determined set of values was the result.

There has been much confusion also as to the possible impact of anyone's set of values on his or her life or professional practice. It can't be claimed, of course, that it is possible to *logically deduce* desired life conduct or educational practice directly from a person's set of values. Nevertheless, it is ridiculous to argue conversely that these values, these presuppositions if you will, do not have a very strong influence on all aspects of a person's life. You, the reader, should keep this distinction firmly in mind as you proceed.

If certain "life values" are available through instruction in some phase of developmental physical activity, whether through gymnasium teaching or athletic coaching, then sincere teacher/coaches should obviously aim to bring about the realization of these values in the lives of their charges. Such values should accordingly become a significant part of the long-range aims of the instructor's personal and professional life. Accordingly, they will presumably also belong to the broader aims of formal and informal education and, somewhat more narrowly, to the aims of physical activity and educational sport either within the educational system or in life outside the school or university.

My plan here, therefore, is to help teachers/coaches *explicitly* assess and develop their underlying set of *implicitly* established personal values. This, then, should provide them with the required "grounding" so they will make the necessary adaptations as they pursue their profession with a reasonable degree of understanding and proficiency. Some fundamental questions will be considered here based largely on the self-evaluation checklist is offered here (see Appendix, p. 230).

Axiology, the fourth subdivision of the discipline of philosophy, is the end result of philosophizing. The individual should strive to develop a system of values reasonably consistent with his or her beliefs in the other three subdivisions as well: metaphysics (or inquiry about the nature of reality); epistemology (or the study of knowledge acquisition); and logic (or the exact relating of ideas). Some believe that values exist only because of the interest of the person who values (*the interest theory*). The *existence theory*, conversely, holds that values exist independently. According to this theory, a person's task is to discover the "real" values, then to give existence to their ideal essence. The *experimental theory* explains values somewhat differently; values that yield results that have "cash value" bring about the possibility of greater happiness through the realization of more effective values in the future. One further theory, the *part whole theory*, postulates that effective relating of appropriate (desired) whole brings about the establishment of the highest values.

Consider next that axiology (the study of values) itself has various domains. First and foremost, we must consider ethics, which has to do with conduct, morality, good and evil, and ultimate objectives in life. There are several approaches to the problem of whether life, as we know it, is worthwhile. A person who goes around with a smile and who looks hopefully toward the future is, of course, an optimist (*optimism*). Some people become easily discouraged and wonder if life is worth the struggle *(pessimism)*. In between these two extremes we find the golden mean, *meliorism* (from the Latin word meaning "better"), which implies that an individual constantly strives to improve his or her situation. This position assumes that the individual cannot make any final decisions about whether good or evil will prevail in the world.

Perhaps the key question to be considered in ethics is, "What is the purpose of *my* existence?" Under this heading we encounter the belief that pleasure is the highest good (*hedonism*). One approach that has developed in modern history from hedonistic doctrine is *utilitarianism*. Here society, not the individual, is the focus, since the basic idea is to promote the greatest happiness for the greatest number of people in the community or world. Although the utilitarian recognizes the existence of various types of pleasure (ranging from intense, momentary emotional pleasure to the pleasure reflected in a placid life based on long-range contentment), he or she believes that seeking this type of pleasure will fulfill the moral duty of life. Another important way of looking at the *summum bonum* (or highest good) in life is called *perfectionism*. Here the individual is aiming for complete self-realization and accordingly envisions someday a society of self-fulfilled people.

A logical outcome of an individual's decision about the greatest good in life is the standard of personal conduct that person sets. Certain interests are apt to guide our conduct. If we are too self-centered, people will say that we are egotistical (*egoism*). Some people go to the other extreme; they feel that a person is best fulfilled by playing down the realization of self-interest in order to serve society or some social group therein (*altruism*). Once again, Aristotle's concept of the golden mean comes to the fore as a workable solution to this question.

One of the other areas of value under axiology deals with the "feeling" aspects of a person's conscious life (*aesthetics*). Aesthetics, the philosophy of taste, asks whether there are principles that govern the search for the beautiful in life. Because there has been a need to define still further values in human life, we now have departmental (specialized) philosophies of religion, education, physical activity education (including sport), etc. Further, we often refer to a person's social philosophy, which simply means that people make decisions about values intrinsic to various institutions.

## Basic Moral Philosophy

In the past, moral philosophers offered general guidance as to what to do, what to seek, and how to treat others--injunctions that we should be fully aware of even today. As a rule, however, philosophers have not tried to preach to their adherents in the same way that theologians have felt constrained to do. These earlier moral philosophers did, however, offer practical advice that included a great variety of pronouncements about what was good and bad, or right and wrong in human life. For example, the terms right and wrong apply only to *acts,* but the terms good and bad refer to (1) the *effects* of acts; (2) the *motives* which caused the act; (3) the *intention* of the person carrying out the act; and (4) the person who is the *agent* of a particular act.

Thus, it might be said correctly that "although Smith is a *good* person, he acted *wrongly*--yet with *good* motives and intentions--when he punched Jones and broke his jaw. The consequences were *bad,* even though Jones had earlier made some threatening gestures at Smith's smaller brother"

Looking back, it can now be appreciated that values, morals, and ethical standards underwent an identity crisis in the 1960s. Since then the pendulum has been swinging back and forth quite violently ever since. Yet, instead of helping society during this period, academic philosophers in North America largely turned their attention to so-called analytic philosophy with its detailed attention to language and related conceptual analysis.

As a result, insight into the human values and morality struggle has devolved to a very small group of philosophers. Conversely the imparting of such insight to "mere mortals" has been assumed by a steadily increasing, much larger group of metaphysical theologians, politicians, playwrights, comedians, and nondescript others. And yet no one can correctly deny the great importance of ethics and human values in people's lives. Nor can the belief be refuted that the question of personal and professional ethics is truly on many people's front burner, but has nevertheless really been in a continuing state of flux for most of the 20th century. It can be argued that the subject is actually so important that it truly demands careful attention at all times.

"Getting in league" with our values is not a simple matter to resolve at any time. People are typically either uncertain or confused on this subject of human values—or conversely they are so strongly indoctrinated that their values seem almost attached to their clothing. Often they may not recognize or accept the fact that they are also confused. Unfortunately, the large majority have quite simply *not* worked out a coherent, consistent, and reasonably logical approach to the values structure that they hold in life.

Further—and it is truly sad—most people simply can't express what it is that they have been working toward in their lives. As it happened "going west", the values that they hold have merely been achieved implicitly and accidentally along the way. They have simply been "handed down" as someone else's or some organization's position, creed, or purpose.

Still further. why is it that—either at home or in our educational system—there has only in rare instance been an opportunity for a person to think this subject through carefully and systematically so that an explicitly determined set of values was the result.

Doesn't it make good sense that today, with problems, conflicts and strife existing at all levels, a person should strive to get to the heart of this vital matter for the sake of his or her future. For several reasons the sad truth is that the child and adolescent in what we call modern society are missing out almost completely on a sound "experiential" introduction to ethics. This has created what may be called an "ethical decision-making dilemma." Frankly, it is a *crisis* and represents a condemnation of present society!

**Meeting the Crisis Directly**

The question is "What to do about this lack?" Where can one go from almost "inherent confusion" that exists in so many lives? The strategy being proposed here for improving this situation is that people should (1) list what they believe our values are in light of the changing times. Then —possibly in discussion with those who are closest to us—they should (2) rearrange and restate them in some type of graduated or hierarchical order.

Thereafter, finally, they will (3) need to assess more carefully--on a regular basis--whether they are living up to those values they have chosen, the values they so often glibly espouse whenever the occasion arises. This bold assertion makes good sense whether reference is being made to what takes place with a person and his or her family in the home, the school, the church, or in the everyday world.

The unpleasant truth is that this lack of an explicit value structure occurs because typically no systematic instruction in this most important subject is offered to a person at any time. Why is this so? One reason is that there are so many different value systems (e.g., religions, societies, advocacy groups) in our society that the educational system shies away from providing such an opportunity. Also, if education authorities were to involve themselves with this subject, these afore-mentioned groups would complain and work to cut off educational funding. Secondly, to become more specific, what evidence is there that people should accept the oft-heard saw that such knowledge is "better caught than taught." Yet, of course, it does helps to have people around you setting good examples. In the final analysis, however, it is the individual alone who, at crucial life-junctures, must make judgments and resultant decisions based on challenges with which he or she is faced.

Having introduced this question broadly, now the next step is to move on to an analysis of the idea of values in people's lives.

## The Values/Ethics Relationship

In the discipline of philosophy, the term "value" is equivalent to the concepts of "worth" and "goodness". It is helpful, however, to draw a distinction between two kinds of value: (1) *intrinsic* value = human experience good or valuable in itself, an end for its own sake, and (2) *extrinsic* value = an experience about goodness or value similarly, while serving as a means to achieve some purpose or material gain.

Ethics is termed a *speculative* subdivision of philosophy that treats the question of values. (Axiology is the technical name for the actual study of values.) It has to do with morality, conduct, good, evil, and the ultimate objectives of life. In discussions one hears such terms as hedonism, perfectionism, egoism, and altruism. As it has developed, there was an ongoing need for people to define values still further in human life. So now there are specialized philosophies of religion, education, art, and even of sport and physical activity education.

The term "ethics" is used in three ways in dictionaries:

(1) To classify a general pattern or "way of life"
(e.g., Muslim ethics)

(2) A listing or rules of conduct or a moral code
    (e.g., professional ethics)
(3) A description of inquiry about ways of life or rules of conduct
    (e.g., that subdivision of ethics known as meta-ethics [e.g.,
    inquiry that treats the meaning and interrelationship of words
    regard as ethical and moral]).

(For example, "What is good and what is bad?" Or "Can standards be
established?" It is in this type of discussion that we encounter the question of
whether values are objective or subjective. In other words, "Do values exist
whether a person is present to realize them or not?" Or "Is it people who ascribe
value to their various relationships with others and their physical environment?")

It can help our understanding to take this question back to the key
philosophers of the early Greek world. Socrates, for example, began the
development of "Western" standards when he recommended the qualities of
goodness, justice, and virtue. Plato, the philosopher who reported this short list to
us, then proceeded to give a spiritual orientation to such thought, believing that
these qualities were timeless--ideas (ideals?) in a world beyond the ken of humans.

Plato was also responsible for suggesting that a mind-body dichotomy might
exist in humans, although–as it turned out–he actually delivered a "mixed
message" in this regard. Conversely, Aristotle, who studied with Plato earlier,
searched for his answers to verities on earth in areas that today are known as the
natural sciences.

It is interesting to note further, however–because it confounds the question
for non-believers in humankind–that St. Thomas Aquinas expanded on Aristotle's
thought--and significantly that of Plato as well. St. Thomas gave humans what has
been called a *spiritual* dimension. He envisioned the human organism as as one
whose make-up includes mind and body--and spirit as well! In the Christian
tradition, however, Catholics subsequently leaned more on Aristotle, whereas
Protestants have identified more with Plato.)

**Ethical Thought Became More Practical**

After the ancient Greeks, ethical thought was oriented more to practice than
to theory. Also, the meanings of ethical terms and concepts did not change
appreciably until marked social change occurred in the 16th and 17th centuries. At

that point it was argued for the first time that ethics should be contrasted with science because the latter was presumably ethically neutral (i.e., value free).

Thereafter, in the Western world at least, a continuing struggle began between advocates of philosophical utilitarianism and those espousing idealism (i.e., the attempt to distinguish between naturalistic ethics and so-called moral law prescribed by some power greater than humans). This struggle has continued to the present day with no firm evidence that it will abate in the near future.

Why is this issue so crucial? The answer seems simple and straightforward because the tendency is to view the matter one way or the other. However, a personal and group decisions made in response to this question will in time no doubt be vital to the future of humans on Earth. As time passes, the enormous ramifications of a decision will necessarily point humankind in one direction or the other.

Looking back to the way that societies developed, the values held by humans became the major social forces that helped to determine the direction a society took at any given moment. The choices made were necessarily based on the values and norms of the culture in which people lived. Such values as *social* values, *educational* values, *scientific* values, *artistic* values, etc. make up the highest level of the social system in a culture. As explained by the brilliant sociologist, Harry M. Johnson (a close colleague of the late, pre-eminent Talcott Parsons), these values when assembled represent the "ideal general character." For example, consider such a value as provision of equality of opportunity to all. In such a setting the overall culture in itself serves a "pattern-maintenance function" as a society confronts the various ongoing "functional problems" it faces (1994).

Throughout history many attempts have been made to define human nature. The values people hold have had a direct relationship as to how the nature of the human being is conceived. Placing them on a historical time scale, Van Cleve Morris (1956) explained that, based on the leading values held at the time, the human has been conceived in five different ways in the history of the Western world as:

(1)     a rational animal
(2)     a spiritual being
(3)     ~~a bundle of impulses~~
(4)     ~~a mind that can be trained by exercise, and~~
(5)     a problem-solving organism (1956)

55

Similarly, Berelson and Steiner (1964) traced six *behavioral-science* images of man and women held throughout recorded history. These images were identified chronologically as:

(1)     the philosophical image
(2)     the Christian image
(3)     the political image
(4)     the economic image, and
(5)     the behavioral-science image

## A Persistent Problem for Humankind: Value Choice

If it is accepted that the values held by people in any particular era are so important, it holds also that the determination of "what is important" has been a "persistent problem" historically for humankind. If an individual or group sought to deviate from what the majority in a society felt about what was important or necessary, a crossroad or crisis in life presented itself. Then, depending on how serious such a problem became, the individual (or group) faced a decision that was either an ethical issue or a legal matter--or both. The society itself determined ultimately what such an "infraction of the rules" was to be called.

Further, as societies evolved, rapidly or slowly, there was greater or lesser confusion about the subject of ethics. The result seems to have been that--instead of having an impossible ideal confronting the practical necessity of daily life–now a vastly diverse inheritance of ethical ways exists. No matter which ethical way of life one chooses, the others "available" are at least to some degree betrayed. This confusion has been exacerbated because of the complex of ethical systems that the West have inherited (i.e., ., Hebraic, Christian, Renaissance, Industrial–and now Islam has been added to the mix!).

What might be termed this "philosophic/religious confusion" has historically and inevitably carried over into all aspects of life. Also, it is probably impossible to gain objectivity and true historical perspective on the rapid change that is taking place. Nevertheless, an unprecedented burden of increasing complexity has been imposed on people's understanding of themselves and their world. Many leaders, along with the rest of the population, must certainly be wondering whether the whole affair can be managed.

Further, the 20th century is said to be one of marked transition from one era to another. Also, some scholars are now beginning to understand that America's blind philosophy of optimism about history's malleability and compatibility in keeping with its ideals may be shortsighted. At least the former weapons stalemate between the U.S.A. and the former U.S.S.R. --not to mention the present "jockeying" between the present leaders--have brought to prominence the importance of non-military determinants (e.g., politics and ideologies).

This fact (i.e., that world peace *must* be maintained) is now sinking into the world's "mentality" especially since there are continuing crises because of the movements toward nuclear-capability expansion by developing powers. Moreover, the world is also witnessing a seemingly inevitable development of a vast ecological crisis that threatens the very existence of life on one small planet known as Earth.

## Leading Philosophical Positions
## Describing Values in the 20th Century

Down through the 20th century, idealism and realism, followed by pragmatism, were the leading philosophical "stances" in the Western world. However, for some scholars what became known as analytic philosophy emanating from England was gradually superseding the "leading stances" in North America. Let us look at each of these positions in this sequence briefly.

*Idealism.* Those holding idealism as their philosophical stance believe the order of the world is due to the manifestation in space and time of an eternal reality. Mind as experienced by all people is basic and real. In fact, the entire universe is essentially mind. The human is more than just a body or an organism. People possess souls, and such possession makes them of a higher order than all other creatures on earth. A soul is an essence of substance that is possessed by a human. It endures after mortal life on Earth is over, Thus, we might say that it is the "vital principle" of an organic body. Some idealists go so far as to believe that this part of the human is also part of God! Since an individual is part of the whole, it is therefore a person's duty to learn as much about the Absolute as possible. Nevertheless, the individual person has freedom to determine which choice he or she will make in life. The individual can relate to the universe's moral law, or else he or she can turn against it.

*Realism.* Those holding realism as their philosophical stance believe that the world exists in itself, apart from our desires and knowledge. There is only one reality—that which we perceive is it. The universe is made up of real substantial entities, existing in themselves and ordered to one another by extra mental relations. Some feel there is one basic unity present, while others holding this position believe in a non-unified cosmos with two or more substances or processes at work. Things don't just happen; they happen because many interrelated forces make them occur in a particular way. People live within this world of cause and effect. They simply cannot make things happen independent of it.

There are two possibilities *religiously* within realism for value achievement in life depending on whether or not the individual realist believes in a Divine Being. For believers, faith and hope would be religious values; for the agnostic or atheist, they would obviously hold little or no value. Wild said that a person may violate the moral law because there is no determinism in that sense (1955, p. 23). However, we must realize that we really don't have complete freedom of choice if we want to lead good lives. This is true, we learn, because laws beyond our control determine thoughts and actions. Broudy said, ". . . to be morally right, therefore, an act must be intended to fill not any claim, but a claim to some good in life." (1961, p. 236)

Religious phenomena are strange things. A great philosopher like Santayana (Durant, 1938, pp. 543-544) found beauty in the ceremony of the Roman Catholic Church, but he did not believe the dogma and denied the possibility of such phenomena. Such phenomena appear to occur universally "in the consciousness which individuals have of an intercourse between themselves and higher powers with which they feel themselves related" (James, 1929, p. 465). It would seem fair to say that realism as a philosophical stance generally takes a middle position (if we may exclude the realism of the Roman Catholic Church for the moment). Perry felt that there was "nothing dispiriting in realism" (1955, p. 347). He saw it as being "opposed equally to an idealistic anticipation of the victory of spirit, and to a naturalistic confession of the impotence of spirit."

*Pragmatism.* Those holding pragmatism as their philosophic position view nature as an emergent evolution. The human's frame of reality is accordingly limited to nature as it functions. The entire world is characterized by activity and change. Through organic evolution rational man and woman have developed over millions of years in this as yet incomplete situation. Humans are confronted by a reality that is constantly undergoing change because a theory of emergent novelty appears to be operating within the universe (multi–verse?). What has proven to be interesting to humankind is that the individual enjoys true freedom of will, a freedom that can be achieved through continuous and developmental learning from experience.

On the basis of this pragmatic philosophic stance, it can be argued that the pragmatic maxim is that the truth or falsehood of a proposition is important only if it has some concrete bearing on the conduct of life for the individual or group. A sharply new assessment of the basic nature of morality seems possible: "A method of integrating (human) impulse and (social) intelligence." This radical deviation from the centuries-old stances could soon lead to the belief that the business of philosophy is to provide a theoretical system that made an integrated whole of our beliefs about the world's nature and the values that humans seek in fulfillment of the nature they have inherited. Presumably, also, humankind has an obligation to advance such an inheritance. As logical as this seemed to many (i.e., the refutation of the traditions of both philosophy and religion), the vested interests of those people being challenged by such pragmatic, "revolutionary" thought have been great indeed.

*Analytic Philosophy*. Early on in the 20th century, small group of philosophers decided to separate itself from the main streams of thought and created another philosophic orientation. This position that we will call "the analytic philosophy movement" gradually deflated and downgraded the long-standing metaphysical and normative types of philosophizing. Accordingly, these centuries-old stances (i.e., idealism and realism) lost much of their basis for justification within the discipline in the 20th century. However, in the Western world, the leading Protestant theologians helped to maintain philosophic idealism, and philosophic realism continued as well because of the under girding it provides for Catholicism.

Nevertheless, the steadily growing population of analytic philosophers moved ahead reasoning that the "wisdom" of their forebears simply could not withstand the rigor of careful analysis. Also, the analytic position seemed to be saying that holding the pragmatic stance with its assessment of the "human condition in a Godless world" was all well and good, but they, the analytic philosophers, had simply come to a different conclusion about their professional task. Accordingly they rejected pragmatism as well as the other two traditional positions.

However, sound theory *is* available to humankind through the application of scientific method to problem-solving. So, in such a case, what then is the exact nature of philosophy? Who is really in a position to answer the ultimate questions about the nature of reality? The scientist is, of course. Accordingly, the philosopher must therefore become the servant of science by the employment of conceptual analysis and rational reconstruction of language to help science develop. The philosopher has no choice but to be resigned to dealing with important, but lesser,

-questions than the origin of the universe, the nature of the human being, and resultant implications for the everyday conduct of this species.

If, therefore, only science and mathematics provide reliable knowledge, philosophy could well then be defined as logical or linguistic analysis. The task of the philosopher accordingly becomes logical or linguistic analysis: the clarification of the meanings of scientific statements. Adoption of this position meant that there were only two kinds of statements: (1) empirical or synthetic statements (e.g., "some metals expand when heated") or (2) analytic statements (e.g., "all circles are squares" as determined by definition). Any other statement a person might wish to make is literally nonsense (i.e., non-sense). Resultantly, it is accordingly non-sense to say that a child is "born in sin," or that a person who has "sinned" according to a religious doctrine that "God will punish you for your sins!".

*Emotivism.* Yet such a strong statement as that does express a strong feeling. One example of this analytic approach resulted in what is called emotivism, a stance where ethical statements would be considered as nothing other than "emotive expression." As the argument goes, such normative statements--being purely emotive--are merely *pseudo-statements*! Such an analytic position argues or explains that a strictly philosophic treatment cannot deal with:

(1) moral exhortation,
(2) descriptions of moral experiences, or
(3) actual value judgments.

If people seek to do this, the result is a pseudo statement that obscures the logical structure of an ethical theory.

Hence,, interestingly, neither subjectivism nor utilitarianism is the answer either. The former, subjectivism, delves into "feelings of approval," an untenable position to base one's future on. The latter, utilitarianism, also tends to look into the psychological state of happiness or pleasure possibly felt by the acceptance of a recommendation of a specific ethical decision.

## How Else Can An Ethical Decision Be Supported?

As the Western world moves into the 21st Century, the matter of values, ethics, and decision-making is more complex than ever. Graham, in his *Eight theories of ethics* (2004), points out that many who seek to enter philosophy's domain are disappointed when they discover that questions about good, evil, and the meaning of life are not answered. Since philosophy's current direction is not so inclined, seeking to ameliorate this dilemma, Graham offers eight theories of, or approaches to, ethics that he views as having stood the test of time. These he identifies as:

(1) egoism,
(2) hedonism,
(3) naturalism & virtue theory,
(4) existentialism,
(5) Kantianism.
(6) utilitarianism,
(7) contractualism, and
(8) religion

In the glossary of *Who Knows What's Right Anymore? (A Guide to Ethical Decision-Making* (Zeigler, 2002), the following definitions of these terms were proposed for the eight extant theories of ethics:

egoism:
The belief that furtherance of the individual's own interests is an acceptable approach for moral action. This motivation of conduct is one of a number of categories under that branch of philosophy known as ethics. It seeks to answer the question as to whether "getting what you want" and the promotion of your own interests is the essence of "the good life."

hedonism:
An ethical doctrine that states humans should guide their ethical conduct on the basis of the personal pleasure such conduct will bring. It should be kept in mind that society has classified the types of personal pleasure into "higher" and "lower" conceptions.

ethical) naturalism & virtue theory
The term "naturalism" describes an early philosophical position that has persisted to the present day. This philosophical theory emphasizes that the physical nature of the universe is self-explanator and denies the presence of any teleological system. The theory called ethical naturalism describes a series of views defined in natural terms. Accordingly, ethical conclusions may be derived from natural objective rules and properties. This stance was popularized by Rousseau and Spencer and subsequently served as a foundation for what has been called progressive education.

existentialism

An approach expressing dissatisfaction with traditional philosophy that is said to have started as a revolt against Hegel's idealism in the latter half of the nineteenth century. It argued that ethical and (what are called) spiritual realities are accessible to humans through reason. In such a world the human's task is to create his/her own essence (i.e., values).

Kantianism

Moral theories developed from the moral philosophy of Ant. He theorized that moral judgment is found "innately" within the rational nature of the human being. People have a "moral" imperative" to do what is right and good in life. They should have to will to carry out such intentions as they seek to gain "immortality" in the way. A "moral action" should be "universally good."

utilitarianism (act and rule)

The belief that the right act for a human is the one that will result in the greatest amount of happiness (net good) in the world. This has subsequently been interpreted as the greatest amount of "intrinsic good" and has also found an interpretation in pragmatic ethics. Some argue that there are two distinct aspects: the heeding and the consequentialist.

contractualism

Moral rationalism is a way to bridge the case between what IS the case and what *ought* to be the case. Morality can be viewed as a set of moral principles with which a society can agree because such as required for ongoing functionality.

religion

The large majority of those subscribing to one of the world's orthodox religions accept that the Deity in one way or another has communicated His will to humans in a variety of ways as to how they should behave on earth. This "religious knowledge" serves as the basis for ethical codes based on human interpretations of God's will..

In bringing this chapter to a close, please consider the challenge that Hunter Lewis issued to humankind in his outstanding treatment of values titled, *A Question of Value* (1990). He stressed that, because of the prevailing confusion and overlap in human thought on the subject, we would be seriously mistaken to consider values "as a Babel that is impossible to make sense of." He concluded:

> Values are *not* the muddle they sometimes seem. There *are* some basic choices, some uniform options that we are all faced with. Our challenge as Americans and as human beings is to identify these options and then to choose among them, not blindly but with a discerning understanding eye, and thus to answer the recurring biblical question: "What manner of men shall we be?" (p. 5).

# Chapter 3
# How Do Humans Choose Values?

Answers to the question posed by the title of Chapter 3 will probably be many and varied. I well recall the confusion engendered 60 years ago when I was invited to be the keynote speaker at a conference of the Ontario Recreation Association. The topic assigned to me was "The Human Values in Recreation." "A great title," I thought, "but how can I get at that topic?

As I recall, at the time I wasn't quite certain exactly what a value was. I knew we spoke glibly about it, but then I asked myself what my own values were. Never having spelled them out with any sort of priority before or *precisely* (!)–and I was age 32 at the time–I thought that such delineation would be helpful as I approached my task. As I recall, determining my own priorities in life in order of importance was "quite an effort and quite an experience." Yet I did it, and then I prepared my talk based on where I thought recreation might conceivably contribute to the achievement of some of my values–and to what extent.

Reflecting on the "happening," if I may call it that, I thought it was strange (significant!) that nowhere in my upbringing, education included, had I gone through such an experience as "listing my personal (life) values in order of importance."

(Parenthetically, I simply can't continue without confessing what the aftermath of my "great speech" was. The president of the provincial association who invited me was a woman serving on the city council in the community where the conference was being held. She rushed up to me, shook my hand and said: "Great speech: What the Hell did you say?" I hope I learned a lesson as a young professional that night...)

Hunter Lewis gives us some help at this point that I wish I had had earlier, back then when I was trying to respond to that "dear lady's" request. In his outstanding treatment of the subject of human values (1990), Lewis stated that there are six ways that people choose the values they hold:

1. Authority (or "I have faith in the authority of...")
2. Deductive Logic ("Since A is true, B must be true. because B follows from A")
3. Sense Experience ("I know it's true because I saw it, I heard it, I tasted it, I smelled it, or I touched it myself.")

4. Emotion ("I feel that this is true.")
5. Intuition ("After struggling with this problem all day, I went to bed confused and exhausted. The next morning, as I awakened, the solution came to me in a flash–and I just knew it was true.")
6. "Science" ("I tested the hypothesis experimentally and found that it was true."

This listing does seem to "cover the waterfront" insofar as individual decision-making is concerned, but then I realized that when to apply which approach is another matter

## Facing a Crisis in Values

So, here we are, individually and collectively facing decisions about "which way to turn" or "what to do about that".  Almost everywhere one turns--there is a crisis in human values as we move along in the 21st century. I believe that most persistent problem that any person faces is the necessity for the ongoing determination (or reaffirmation) of his or her values. We all hold such values necessarily as part of our background experience.

In addition, I believe there are actually three categories into which these values may be divided:

First, those which are personal in the sense that they relates to our immediate relations with family and friends--and our everyday life in society functioning under this or that social or political system.

Secondly, as we become professionals in some field of endeavor, we should also explicitly determine our professional value orientation as a fundamental aspect of our relationship to the clients that we serve.

Then, thirdly, because of the way the world seems to be going, we are faced with the determination of our social or environmental values. The world is becoming ever-more precarious--and "it's getting real scary out there!"

All of this is not a simple matter to resolve. People are often confused and uncertain in this regard, but frequently they may not recognize or accept the fact that they are confused.  Seemingly they simply have not worked out a coherent, consistent, and reasonably logical approach to the values that they hold–or think they hold–in life. Most people simply can't express what it was they are working toward in their lives. Typically their values that they held had been achieved *implicitly* and accidentally along the way. Usually they have simply been "handed" down as someone's or some organization's position, creed, or purpose. Only in rare instances has an opportunity been provided for them to think this subject through carefully and systematically so an *explicitly* determined set of values was present for them to bring to bear in decision-making.

In my books *Who Knows What's Right Anymore? and Whatever Happened to "the Good Life?"* (2002), as well as in *A Way Out of Ethical Confusion* (2004), I strove to get to the heart of this massive problem in different ways. I argued that, for several reasons, the child and adolescent in society today are missing out almost completely on a sound "experiential" introduction to ethics. I believe this has created what I call an "ethical decision-making dilemma."

## What Should Happen to Correct This Situation?

We need to reconsider *our* values and then re-state **IN SOME TYPE OF GRADUATED OR HIERARCHICAL ORDER** –i.e., exactly what we believe they are in light of the changing times, and then, finally, we will then need to assess more carefully--on a regular basis--whether we are living up to those values we have chosen and so often glibly espouse.

This is true whether we are referring to what takes place in the home, the school system, the church**, OR OUT IN THE EVERYDAY WORLD.** The truth is that typically no systematic instruction in this most important subject is offered at any time. (And I refuse to accept the often-heard "osmosis stance"--that such knowledge is "better caught than taught.") It helps to have people around you who are setting good examples.

However, *in the final analysis it's the individual who makes judgments and decisions based on experiences undergone.*

## How Values Have Been Viewed Historically

1. Socrates began the development of Western standards when he considered the qualities of goodness, justice, and virtue.

66

2. Plato followed by giving a type of "spiritual" orientation to such thought. He believed ta these qualities were timeless–ideas (ideals?) in a world beyond the ken of man.
3. Aristotle, Plato's student, searched conversely for his answers on earth in what have become the *natural* sciences.

> **Note:** Interestingly, St. Thomas Aquinas picked up on Aristotle's work by giving it a spiritual dimension (i.e., spirit, mind, and body). Catholics have resultantly leaned more on Aristotle, whereas Protestants jave identified more with Plato.

After the ancient Greeks, ethical thought was oriented more to practice than to theory. The meanings ethical terms and concepts did not change appreciably until marked social change in the 16th and 17th centuries. At that point it was argued that ethics should be contrasted with science because the latter was presumably ethically neutral (i.e., value free).

Thereafter began a continuing struggle between utilitarianism and idealism (i.e., the attempt to distinguish between naturalistic ethics and moral law). The latter possibly prescribed by some power greater than humans).

## Ethics in Philosophy

Here the term "value" is equivalent to the concepts of "worth" and "goodness".

> **Note:** It is helpful here to draw a distinction between two kinds of value (1) *intrinsic* value = human experience good or valuable in itself, and end for its own sake, and (b) *extrinsic* value = an experience that brings about goodness of value similarly, while serving as a means to achieve some purpose or material gain.

Since ethics is a (speculative) subdivision of philosophy that treats the question of values (i.e., having to do with morality, conduct, good, evil, and ultimate objectives in life), we hear suc terms as hedonism, perfectionism, egoism, and altruism.

Because there is a need to define values still further in life, we now have specialized philosophies of religion, education, education, physical activity education (including sport), etc.

## Axiology (The Study of Values)

The term ethics is used in three ways:

(1) To classify a "way" or pattern of life (e.g., Muslim ethics
(2) A listing of rules of conduct that is often called a moral code
(e.g., professional ethics)
3) A description of an investigation or inquiry about rules of
conduct or a way of life (e.g., a subdivision of ethics termed
meta-ethics = inquiry that treats the meaning and
interrelationship of words viewed as moral and ethical.

For example, what is right or wrong; good or bad? Once again, we encounter the question of whether values are objective or subjective (i.e., do values exist whether a person is present to realize them or not? Or, for example, is it people who ascribe value to this or that relationship with others or with their physical environment?

We might ask: "Why is it so important that people give consideration to the topic of values in their lives?" The answer is that values are the major social forces that help to determine the direction a culture will take at any given moment. Choices made are necessarily based on the values and norms of the culture in which people live. Such values, social values, educational values, scientific values, artistic values, etc., make up the highest level of the social system in a culture. These values represent the "ideal general character" (e.g., social-structured facilitation of individual achievement, equality of opportunity). Remember that overall culture in itself also serves a "pattern-maintenance function" as a society confronts the ongoing functional problems it faces.

Further, the values people hold have a direct relationship to how the nature of the human being is conceived. A number of attempts have been made to define human nature on a rough historical time scale. For example, the human has been conceived in five different ways in historical progression as (1) a rational animal, (2) a spiritual being, (3) a receptacle of knowledge, (4) a mind that can be trained by exercise, and (5) a problem-solving organism (Morris, 1956). Likewise, Berelson and Steiner (1964) traced six behavioral-science images of man and woman throughout recorded history. Identified chronologically they are: (1) a philosophical image, (2) a Christian image, (3) a political image, (4) an economic image, (5) a psychoanalytic image, and (6) a behavioral-science image.

## The "Persistent Problem" of Values Has Brought Confusion?

As explained previously rapid change in society had caused general confusion about the subject of ethics. Instead of having an impossible ideal confronting the practical necessity of daily life, we have such a diverse inheritance of ethical ways that no matter which one we choose, the others are at least to some degree betrayed. Obviously, this confusion has been exacerbated because of the complex of moral systems that we have inherited (e.g., Hebraic, Christian, Renaissance, Industrial--and now Islam too, for example).

This confusion philosophic/religious confusion has historically carried over into all aspects of life. Today, it may well be impossible to gain objectivity and true historical perspective on the rapid change that is taking place. Nevertheless, a seemingly unprecedented burden of increasing complexity has been imposed on people's understanding of themselves and their world. Many leaders, along with the rest of us, must certainly be wondering whether the whole affair can be managed.

Further, as we now comprehend that the 20th century was indeed one of marked transition from one era to another, some scholars are beginning to understand that America's quite blind philosophy of optimism about history's malleability and compatibility in keeping with North American ideals may turn out to be very shortsighted. At least the weapons stalemate between the U.S.A. and the former U.S.S.R. brought to prominence the importance of nonmilitary determinants (e.g., politics and ideologies). This fact has--and also has **NOT**--sunk into the world's mentality. Most importantly, the world is witnessing the gradual, but seemingly inevitable, development of a vast ecological crisis that threatens the very existence of the planet known as Earth.

## The Basic Question: How Do People Choose Values?

Keeping everything that has been said here in mind, generally speaking, how *do* people emerge from what appears to be an absolute muddle when it comes to choosing their values in their lives? Are there some commonalities? What are the options available to us?

Fortunately I was able to turn for help at this point to the outstanding book by Hunter Lewis (1990) titled *a question of values*. Lewis asks whether humans have "freely chosen values" over and above the inherited instincts that drive us all daily because of out inherited genes. He opines that freely chosen values do indeed supplement our basic instincts, In fact he believes that at times they completely supplant this or that instinct. In other words, without freely chosen values we would probably have self-destructed eons ago.

This brings us back to the basic question as to how we arrive at our beliefs. We are exhorted to make a list of our beliefs and then to ask ourselves exactly why as an individual I chose to implement this or that belief in my life. Lewis did this and eventually decided upon a list delineating six ways available to humans as follows:

1. Authority:         Taking someone else's word
2. Deductive Logic:   Applying deductive reasoning
3. Sense experience:  Getting knowledge from one
                      of our five senses
4. Emotion:           Feeling that something is right
5. Intuition:         Using unconscious, but rational– thought
6. "Science":         Using a technique relying on
                      facts, logic, and testable hypotheses

## The Dilemma Faced by All

Keeping the above six ways recommended by Lewis firmly in mind, in my teaching of ethical decision making, I finally adopted a three-step or "trivium" approach used by Prof. Richard Fox at Cleveland State University for 30 years as an initial approach to get his students started.

Proceeding on the assumption that a professional person should be able to work out rationally what right and wrong ethical behavior is, he recommended an approach in which there is a progression from the thought of Kant, to Mill, and then to Aristotle.  This mat be called a "three-step approach" (or a "trivium" and consists of the application of three "tests" (phrased as questions) to be applied when one wishes to analyze an ethical problem or dilemma.

*The three tests*:
    (1) the test of consistency, or universalizability;
    (2) the test of consequences; and
    (3) the test of intentions.

I concur with Professor Fox that all people should have an initial experiences in ethical decision-making as they strive to develop their value systems related to the personal, professional, and social or environmental aspects of their lives. I believe this three-step approach can be used profitably by anyone in all aspects or dimensions of his/her life. In other words, whether the decision-making has to do with the personal, professional, or social/environmental aspects of that person's life.

*An example: "Everybody's Doin' It".* Brad, a college graduate in business administration, obtained a position with responsibility for assisting with the advertising and marketing of his firm's products. His superior, Wesley, appeared to be a real "go-getter." One of the people in the marketing department described him as a person who "wanted to start at the top and work up." Nevertheless, Wes seemed to want to be very helpful to Brad in a number of different ways. Brad was anxious to do well with his new job, of course, and he appreciated the fact that someone was willing to "show him the ropes." As time passed, however, Brad began to perceive that he and Wes were really operating on different wave lengths (so to speak). He told Barbara, his wife, that Wes was really much more realistic and pragmatic than he was. Wes was always trying to cut corners and to get ahead of the other guy (the firm's competitors or even the consumer for that matter). "I guess I'm just too idealistic," Brad said to Barbara one evening during dinner, "but in writing advertising copy I try to tell the truth about our products. They are good, of that I'm certain, but Wes is always on me to write what I feel is dishonest, 'borderline,' fraudulent copy." On Barbara's urging, Brad invited Wes out for a beer after work and explained his concerns to him. Wes replied that he knew what Brad was talking about, and he also said that he felt that way once too. "But," he concluded, "I soon learned that the only to get there is to be as 'borderline' as everyone else in this business. It's 'dog-eat-dog' out there, and you simply have to cheat a little here and there and occasionally make wild claims that may not be true--or you'll be left behind in the dust." How should Brad cope with this situation?

*Analysis.* On the surface the problem faced by Brad seems pretty much "black and white"; either you practice honesty or not. However, as many of us learn along the way, this question can be a highly complex one in numerous life situations encountered. Human relations at the personal level and at the professional level are rarely simple. It is an unfortunate fact that a significant minority of the populace seem to be ready to cheat or be dishonest in small ways--and at times in more serious ways as well. Then these people of questionable morality tend to rationalize their actions by saying, "Oh, everybody does it, so why shouldn't I?" T permit even minor dishonesty as a "standard" of virtue, either in personal or professional life would be fundamentally wrong .

In addition, if we apply Kant's principle of universality to this matter, it is obvious that everyone doesn't cheat and be dishonest.

Secondly, just think of what the net consequences of "everyone doing it" (Mill's principle) would be. It would obviously not be a very nice world in which to live.

Lastly, are there situations (Aristotle's thought) where you might be dishonest and yet be moral? Probably very few, although every day we do run into the so-called "white lie" where you may be dishonest in a sense that you lie to someone because you don't want to hurt his or her feelings. And it is true, of course, that a great many people are dishonest in business with their marketing practices when they practice what I call the "We're the greatest!" syndrome even if they know they aren't--if the truth be told. To return to the case at hand, it appears that Brad is going to have to engage in a large measure of soul-searching if he is going to continue and be successful in his present position.

## Some Final Thoughts on Becoming a Person Holding Wise Values

A twenty-first century person has a choice to make. He or she must think deeply about the philosophic/religious position he or she holds has validity in the world of the 21st century.

If this person's position leads to the adoption of one of the world's great religions. it would seem vital that he or she should really follow through with the dictates of their particular faith.

It would seem to be crucial, however, that the leaders of the various world religions must work for consensus wherever possible on the great issues confronting humankind. Otherwise the perennial confrontations will only lead to frustration and eventual disaster.

I have personally come to believe that the world's religions are myths that have outlived their usefulness. I believe they are probably doing more harm than good through the conflicts they have engendered in the past and at present--and will continue to exacerbate in the future.

My own approach is "pragmatic" in the sense that I do not see the universe as having built-in values. I believe that humans should create their own values in an ever-changing world. As part of the process, I think they should then establish a priority with their values to help put their individual lives in perspective in a changing world.

Finally, I want to reiterate:

(1) In many ways we are confused about what our values are at the present,
(2) We need to reconsider them and then re-state exactly what we believe they are in light of the changing times, and
(3) Finally, we will then need to assess more carefully--on a regular basis--whether we are living up to those values we have chosen and so often glibly espouse.

# Chapter 4
## What Is the Function of Value in Society?

### The General External Environment

It is not always possible to state definitively where the immediate (internal) environment leaves off and the general (external) environment begins in a given society. All known societies are open systems, often involving a variety of subgroups within their geographical boundaries. Careful definition of a particular society is a highly complex task, each one having certain unique qualities while undoubtedly possessing many similarities with other societies. The components of societies are usually described as subsystems (e.g., the economy, the government). In a very real sense these subsystems have been developed to "divide up the work," and it is with the interweaving of these systems that the remainder of this section will be concerned. We must keep in mind here that the larger society, here discussed first, is infinitely more complex than any organization that exists within it. However, it is important to be reminded that many of the concepts and group roles of the society can be transferred from one societal level to the other (and vice versa).

### General Action System Has Four Subsystems

Before considering a more general discussion of the external environment from the standpoint of resources, the various social organizations, the power structure, and the value structure, there will be a relatively brief presentation of Parsonsian "Action Theory." This particular (grand) theory has a long tradition in the field of sociology. It has been described by Johnson (1969; 1994)--to whom this book is dedicated--as being "a type of empirical system" that actually applies to an extremely wide range of systems from relationships between two people to that of total societies. It cannot be regarded as totally concerned with economic theory; it is more "a generalization of economics." It seeks to analyze both structure and process.

Initially, to understand this social theory, a person should appreciate that the general action system (implying instrumental activism) is viewed as being composed of four subsystems: (a) cultural system, (b) social system, (c) psychological system, and (d) behavioral-organic system. What this means, viewed from a different perspective, is that explicit human behavior is comprised of aspects that are cultural, social, psychological, and organic. These four subsystems together compose a cybernetic hierarchy of control and conditioning that operates in both

74

directions (i.e., both up and down). (Johnson [1994] explains that an example of a cybernetic system might be a thermostat and an air-conditioning unit [p. 57] . . . . there is an "instrumental activism" occasioned by the "value pattern" of modern societies in which a person' self esteem depends on the extent a contribution is made in some way to life's advancement.)

The reader might already be aware of the general ideas within social theory that explain primary and secondary control in society, but this person might not understand specifically that Parsons contribution (his innovation!) to this theory is the application of cybernetics to what has become known as the L-I-G-A four functional categories proceeding from the most controlling level, L, to the least controlling, A. These terms may be used as variables in Parsons' formal paradigm that can be employed systematically to assist in the functional analysis of of what Johnson (1994) calls "an indefinite large number of empirical problems" (p. 58).

The first of the subsystems is "culture," which according to Johnson (1969) "provides the figure in the carpet-the structure and, in a sense, the 'programming' for the action system as a whole" (p. 46). The structure of this type of system is typically geared to the functional problems of that level that  arise--and so on down the scale, respectively. Thus it is the subsystem of culture that legitimates and also influences the level below it (the social system). Typically, there is a definite strain toward consistency. However, the influence works both upward and downward within the action system, thereby creating a hierarchy of influence or conditioning.

Social life being what it has been and is, it is almost inevitable that strain will develop within the system. Johnson explains this as "dissatisfaction with the level of effectiveness on the functioning of the system in which the strain is felt" (p. 47). Such dissatisfaction may, for example, have to do with particular aspects of a social system as follows: (1) the level of effectiveness of resource procurement; (2) the success of goal attainment; (3) the justice or appropriateness of allocation of rewards or facilities; or (4) the degree to which units of the system are committed to realizing (or maintaining) the values of the system.

Strain may arise at the personality or psychological system level, and the resultant pressure could actually change the structure of the system above (the social system). This is not inevitable, however, because such strain might well be resolved satisfactorily at its own level (so to speak). Usually the pattern consistency
of the action system display reasonable flexibility, and this is especially true at the lower levels. For example, strain might be expressed by deviant behavior or in

other ways such as by reduced identification with the social system by the person or group concerned.

Thus, it is the hierarchy of control and conditioning that comes into play when the sources of change (e.g., new religious or scientific ideas) begin to cause strain in the larger social systems, whereas the smaller social systems tend to be "strained" by the change that often develops at the personality or psychological system levels. In addition, it is quite apparent that social systems are often influenced considerably by contact with other social systems.

## Levels of Structure
## Within the Social System

Just as there were four subsystems within the total action system defined by Parsons and others, there are evidently four levels within the subsystem that has been identified as the social system or structure. These levels, proceeding from "highest" to "lowest," are (1) values, (2) norms, (3) the structure of collectivities, and (4) the structure of roles. Typically the higher levels are more general than the lower ones, with the latter group giving quite specific guidance to those segments or units of the particular system to which they apply. These "units" or "segments" are either collectivities or individuals in their capacity as role occupants.

*Values* represent the highest echelon of the social system level of the entire general action system. These values may be categorized into such "entities" as artistic values, educational values, social values, sport values, etc. Of course, all types or categories of values must be values of personalities. The social values of a particular social system are those values that are conceived of as representative of the ideal general character that is desired by those who ultimately hold the power in the system being described. The most important social values in North America, for example, have been (1) the rule of law, (2) the socio-structural facilitation of individual achievement, and (3) the equality of opportunity (Johnson, 1969, p. 48).

*Norms* are the shared, sanctioned rules which govern the second level of the social structure. The average person finds it difficult to separate in his or her mind the concepts of values and norms. Keeping in mind the examples of values offered immediately above, some examples of norms are (1) the institution of private property, (2) private enterprise, (3) the monogamous, conjugal family, and (4) the separation of church and state.

*Collectivities* are interaction systems that may be distinguished by their goals, their composition, and their size. A collectivity is characterized by conforming acts and by deviant acts, which are both classes of members' action which relate to the structure of the system. Interestingly (and oddly) enough, each collectivity has a structure that consists of four levels also (not discussed here). In a pluralistic society one finds an extremely large variety of collectivities that are held together to a varying extent by an overlapping membership constituency. Thus, members of one collectivity can and do exert greater or lesser amounts of influence upon the members of the other collectivities to which they belong.

*Roles* refer to the behavioral organisms (the actual humans) who interact within each collectivity. Each role has a current normative structure specific to it, even though such a role may be gradually changing. (For example, the role of the sport manager or physical activity educator/coach or recreation director could be in a transitory state in that certain second-level norms could be changing, and yet each specific sport manager (or physical educator/coach or recreation director) still has definite normative obligations that are possible to delineate more specifically than the more generalized second-level norms, examples of which were offered above.)

*A hierarchy of control and conditioning.* Finally, these four levels of social structure themselves also compose *a hierarchy of control and conditioning*. As Johnson (p. 49) explains, the higher levels "legitimate, guide, and control" the lower levels, and pressure of both a direct and indirect nature can be--and generally is--employed when the infraction or violation occurs and is known.

## Functional Interchanges

A society is the most nearly self-subsistent type of social system and, interestingly enough again, societies or "live systems or personalities" typically have four basic types of functional problems (each with its appropriate value principle) as follows:

1. A pattern-maintenance problem (**L**) that has to do with the inculcation of the value system and the maintenance of the social system's commitment to it,
2. An integration problem (**I**) that is at work to implement the value of solidarity expressed through norms that accordingly regulate the great variety of processes

3. A goal-attainment problem (**G**) that implements the value of effectiveness of group or collective action on behalf of the social system toward this aim, and

4. An adaptation problem (**A**) whereby the economy implements the value of utility (i.e., the investment-capitalization unit). (See Figure 1 below).

The economy of a society is its adaptive subsystem, while the society's form of government (polity) has become known as its goal-attainment subsystem. The integrative and pattern-maintenance subsystems, which do not have names that can be used in everyday speech easily, consist actually of a set or series of processes by which a society's production factors are related, combined, and transformed with utility-the value principle of the adaptive system-as the interim product. These products "packaged" as various forms of "utility" are employed in and by other functional subsystems of the society.

Thus, each subsystem exchanges factors and products, becomes involved as pairs, and engages in what has been called a "double interchange." It is theorized that each subsystem contributes one factor and one product (i.e., one category or aggregate of factors and one category or aggregate of products) to each of the other three functional subsystems. Considered from the standpoint of all the pairs possible to be involved in the interchange, there are therefore six double-interchange systems. Factors and products are both involved in the transformational processes, each being functional for the larger social system. Factors are general and therefore more remote, while products are specific and therefore more directly functional. The performance of the functional requirements has been described as a "circular flow of interchanges," with the factors and products being continuously used up and continuously replaced.

An example of interchange process taking place begins to help us see how this complex circular flow of interchanges occurs. Johnson explains how one of the six interchange systems functions typically to create the political support system in a society. This is how the functional problem of goal-attainment is resolved through the operation of the society's form of government (polity)--that is, the interchange between the polity and the integrative subsystems. "The political process is the set of structured activities that results in the choice of goals and the mobilization of societal resources for the attainment of these goals" (p. 51). First, the integrative system contributes to political accomplishment by achieving

FIGURE 1

THE FUNCTIONAL PROBLEMS OF SOCIAL SYSTEMS*

|  | Instrumental | Consummatory |
|---|---|---|
| INTERNAL | **(L)**<br>**LATENT**<br>**PATTERN MAINTENANCE**<br>**& TENSION MANAGEMENT**<br><br>(Involves Stability &<br>Continuity in Relations<br>Among Units) | **(I)**<br><br>**INTEGRATION**<br><br><br>(Involves Success &<br>Satisfaction in Inter-<br>Unit Relationships) |
| EXTERNAL | **(A)**<br>**ADAPTATION**<br><br>(Involves Stability &<br>Continuity in<br>Relation to External<br>Environment) | **(G)**<br>**GOAL-ATTAINMENT**<br><br>(Involves Success &<br>Satisfaction in<br>Relation to External<br>Environment) |

*Adapted from Johnson, H.M. (1994). Modern organizations in the Parsonsian theory of action. In A. Farazmand (Ed.), *Modern organizations: Administrative theory in contemporary society* (p. 59). Westport, CT: Praeger; and Hills, R.J. (1968). *Toward a science of organization* (p. 21). Eugene, OR: Center for Advanced Study of Administration.

a certain degree of consensus and "solidarity." These qualities are "registered" and "delivered" in the form of votes and interest demands. These are, in fact, forms of political support-that is, support from the integrative system to the polity. Conversely, in return, the government (polity) bolsters (integrative) solidarity through political leadership that, in turn, produces binding decisions. Thus, this leadership and the binding decisions can also be considered as "political support"-- support from the polity or government to the integrative system (one of the two systems that "produces utility"--i.e., implements one of the four values of which utility is one.)

## The Social Significance of Interchange Analysis

As can be seen from the example given above, the interchange analysis has tremendous social significance. The interchange of factors and products identifies the types of processes that somehow must take place in any social system. This scheme specifies also their functional significance and also indicates relations between these processes that are broad but yet important. As was stated earlier, the functional subsystems compose a hierarchy of control and conditioning. Thus, the processes involved are influenced, conditioned, and controlled. These same interchange processes must be going on in any functioning social system, but it should be understood that their specific forms vary greatly. The four levels of a particular social system (i.e., values, norms, collectivities, roles) provide the forms and channels by which any unique social system carries on its functionally necessary processes. Fundamental social change means that some basic transformation has taken, or is taking, place in one or more levels of the social system (structure). Obviously, basic change must inevitably affect the operation of the system in some distinct, measurable way.

The social change that may take place within a social system can be viewed as one of three types--i.e., one of three levels of analysis that may be distinguished as follows: (1) the analysis of "circular flow," which explains the pattern of interchange process occurring within a stable social system; (2) the analysis of "growth patterns," which determines the growth or decline of particular attributes or products of the system (e.g., power, wealth); and (3) the analysis of structural change, which is the determination of whether a level or levels of the system undergo any substantive change due to strong lower-level strain.

Critics of such social theory (here defined as Parsonsian) seem to overlook the fact that it makes definite allowance for equilibrium and change; in fact, radical social change, with or without an actual revolution, does institute a new hierarchy

80

of control and conditioning. This occurs, for example, when the strain at the three lower levels forces a different set of priorities in the value subsystem. These new values become resultantly the basic source of legitimization, guidance, and control for the levels below.

Parsons' general action system is then actually an "equilibrium model," but this does not mean that it is necessarily conservative and/or static. As explained above, social systems may, or may not, be in a state of equilibrium, and change is certainly most possible within this theory's framework. This theory is a reasonable, theoretical explanation of how social change can and does take place. Social systems are conceived of as having a normative structure, which may or may not be stable. To understand how to achieve equilibrium within a social system, it is at least theoretically necessary to learn to distinguish between processes that will maintain or change a given social structure. Finally, it is important to understand that sometimes the higher levels of social structure may be maintained (if this is desired and desirable) by understanding how to change one or more of its lower levels. Quite obviously, this last point is most important to anyone serving in a managerial capacity in any organization within a given social system.

The above brief discussion of some of the basic elements of developing Parsonsian theory of action has necessarily avoided the introduction of this information in great detail. For example, the concepts of economic theory involved in the adaptive subsystem of a society (i.e., money, utility, products, and factors of production) were not presented. Such presentation would help the reader to appreciate their close counterparts in the theory of the other three functional problems of social systems (e.g., goal-attainment).

Nor has there been any discussion of the idea, presented by Parsons, that any analysis of the structure of complex societies demands careful differentiation of four levels of organizations (not considered as an entity). These levels have been called the technical, managerial, institutional, and societal levels, and it is clear that these four primary-level outputs are closely related to the four functional problems described above. Technical-level systems involving small groups of people using facilities and making decisions must be coordinated with the managerial level of organizations--and so on up the scale through the regulation of institutionalized norms until the societal level is reached where the "single focus" of first-order values is brought to bear on the operation. (This differentiation of organizational levels is discussed below under the "application to organizations" section because of its direct relationship to the managerial function.)

Still further, the symbolic media of society have not been introduced (generalized commitments, influence, power, and money), and they are fundamentally important to the understanding and operation of the four basic types of subsystems within a social system as explained through the functional problems that have been technically identified as pattern-maintenance, integration, goal-attainment, and adaptation.

These "actors" and others of an even more technical nature must be mastered by someone who truly wished to specialize in what might be called the general or external environment, but it was felt that what has been presented is sufficient to introduce managers generally to a basic understanding of the general environment.

# Chapter 5
# The Value Attached to Human Physical Activity
# (including Sport) in World History

## Brief Historical Background

*Primitive and Preliterate Societies.* In primitive society there was probably very little organized purposive instruction in developmental physical activity in sport, exercise, and related expressive movement; any incidental education was usually a byproduct of daily experience. The usual activities of labor, searching for food, rhythmic activities, and games were essential to the development of superior bodies. Physical education activities, in addition to promoting physical efficiency, helped to strengthen membership in the society and served also as a means of recreation.

*China.* In the ancient Chinese civilization, formal physical training and organized sport presumably had little if any place in a culture whose major aim was to preserve and perpetuate a traditional social order. At that time no strong military motive existed, although physical training was used sporadically when it did become necessary to increase military efficiency. As a type of classical education grew and various religious influences were felt, even less emphasis was placed on formal physical development, and health standards were poor indeed. In later Chinese history the value of training to bear arms was appreciated much more because of the changing nature of the type of combat in which the men engaged.

*India.* In ancient India, the climate and religious philosophy forced a relative rejection of physical training for all save the ever-present dancing girls of the ancient world. Further, those men in the military caste were trained physically to bear arms in defense of their society. Certain hygienic rules and ritualistic dances were common to the Hindus, but typically they were connected with religious ceremonies.

*Egypt* In early Egypt also, physical training was not part of the typical educational system, although as in the other early cultures the average person, male or female, did receive a greater or lesser amount of exercise depending upon his or her daily work regimen. As the social life grew in complexity and a class structure developed, the upper class received a level of education that was not available to the great majority of people. Sports, games, and dancing were popular with the nobility, the latter activity being included in religious life for common people as well.

*Babylon and Assyria.* The Tigris-Euphrates civilization did not seem to give physical education much status either, except for the perennial warrior class and for those occupations that demanded varying levels of physical fitness for their adequate execution.

*Israel.* The Hebrews promoted certain physical activities and hygienic practices mainly because of the influence of their religious heritage and their desire to preserve their national unity, but it may not be assumed that they valued physical education highly for all. Later, under the influence of the Greeks and then the Romans, their attitude changed in certain locales. However, sports were never popular among <u>all</u> Hebrews of the ancient world.

*Persia.* In contrast, the Persians rivaled ancient Greece in many of its methods of physical training. Physical fitness was very valuable to them because it served to produce the stamina needed for great armies. They went to extremes in developing excellent hunters, horsemen, and warriors. However, their concept of physical education was very narrow because of their desire for military supremacy.

*Greece.* Physical education and athletic games were valued very highly in ancient Greek society. From 1100 to 700 B.C., the Homeric Age, athletic games held a prominent place. The aim of physical education was to produce a man of action, and great concern was shown for individual excellence. The well-rounded man-citizen-soldier was the ideal, a person who steadily increased in wisdom as well. The *Spartan* Greeks were almost completely concerned with the development of devoted citizens and outstanding soldiers or warriors. They placed great stress upon almost unbelievably difficult physical training and hardship as part of the training at arms; the end product was an almost invincible soldier in single combat. Athletics were not considered important unless they contributed directly to soldierly prowess. *Athenian* Greeks also valued physical education most highly for its contribution to the development of the ideal individual. However, the harmonious development of body and soul (mind) was of paramount concern. Although such overall development was available only to free men in a society where slaves were ordinarily obtained and then kept because of military victories, there has probably never been another culture--if this city-state may be so designated--in which the development of the all-round citizen was more cherished. In later Athenian Greece, as the society became more complex and was conquered by Rome, gradually increasing emphasis was placed on intellectual excellence; the majority of youth lost interest in excellent physical development, and eventually extreme professionalism in athletics grew to such an extent that the former ideal was lost forever.

*Rome.* The Romans were much more utilitarian in their attitude toward physical training; they simply did not grasp the concept of the Greek ideal. They valued physical training for very basic reasons: it developed a man's knowledge in the skills of war, and it kept him healthy because of the strict regimen required. It helped to give a man strength and endurance and made him courageous in the process. Later in Roman history as the army became more specialized, the value of physical training for all became less apparent, although it was still practiced by most citizens to a degree for the maintenance of health and for recreational pursuits. Athletic festivals and fierce games in the arena, often of a highly barbaric nature, were held regularly for the entertainment of the masses in order to gain political support for the various office holders.

*Visigoths.* The Visigoths ("visi" means east) began their successful invasions to the south about 376 A.D., and the end of the Roman Empire has usually been designated as 100 years later (476 A.D.). The period following has been commonly called, but now seemingly incorrectly thought of as, the "Dark Ages," a time when most literature and learning came to a standstill and might have been completely lost save for the newly organized monasteries. "Ill blows the wind that profits nobody" is a proverb that applies to this era. The Visigoths did possess abundant energy and splendid bodies and are presumed to have helped the virility of the civilized world of the West at that time. The Moslem leader Tarik ended the Visigoth kingdom in 711 in the battle at Guadalete.

As the immoral society of the declining Romans became a mere memory, Christianity continued to spread because of the energy, enthusiasm, and high moral standards of its followers. The Church managed to survive the invasion of the barbarians and gradually became an important influence in the culture, and its continued growth seemed a certainty. Although the historic Jesus Christ in many ways was said to be anything but an ascetic, the early Christians perverted history to a degree as they envisioned the individual's moral regeneration as the highest goal. They became most concerned with their souls and the question of eternal happiness. (It should be pointed out that with the Greeks it was a mind or soul and body dichotomy, but that St. Thomas Aquinas later added the dimension of soul or spirit to the mind and body dichotomy and made the human a tripartite creature.) Matters of the body were presumed to be of this world, and consequently of Satan;

85

affairs of the soul were of God. This way of life has been given the name of asceticism, the main idea being to subdue the desires of the flesh--even by torture if necessary.

The belief has prevailed that most churchmen were opposed to the idea of physical education or training, but this has been called "The Great Protestant Legend" (Ballou, 1965). On balance it does seem more logical that these Christians would not be opposed to the idea of hard work and strenuous physical activity, but that they would indeed be violently opposed to all types of sports, games, and athletic festivals associated with earlier pagan religions and the horrible excesses of the Roman arena and hippodrome. And so for hundreds of years during the period known as the Early Middle Ages, physical education, as it is known today, found almost no place within the meager educational pattern that prevailed, a very sterile period indeed for those interested in the promulgation of physical education and sport of the finest type. Eventually even much of the physical labor in the fields and around the grounds of the monasteries was transferred to nonclerics. Thus, even this basic physical fitness was lost to this group as more intellectual pursuits became the rule. As is so often the case, the pendulum had swung too far in the other direction.

*Feudalism* or *Age of Chivalry* Physical training was revived to a degree in the period known as the Age of Chivalry. Feudal society was divided into three classes: (1) the masses, who had to work to support the other classes and to eke out a bare subsistence for themselves; (2) the clergy, who carried on the affairs of the Church; and (3) the nobles, who were responsible for the government of certain lands and territories under a king, and who performed military duties. During this time a physical and military education of a most strenuous type was necessary along with a required training in social conduct for the knight who was pledged to serve his feudal lord, the Church, and, presumably, all women as well as his own lady in particular. Such an ideal was undoubtedly better in theory than in practice, but it did serve to set standards higher than those which existed previously. The aim of physical training was certainly narrow according to today's ideal, and understandably health standards were typically very poor. The Greek ideal had been forgotten, and physical education once again served a most practical objective: to produce a well-trained individual in the art of hand-to-hand combat with all of the necessary physical attributes such as strength, endurance, agility, and coordination. With the subsequent invention of machinery of war, the enemy was not always met at close range. As a result, death in battle became to a larger extent accidental and was not necessarily the result of physical weakness and ineptitude in warfare techniques. Naturally, some divergence took place in the aims and methods of military training and allied physical training.

Just before the Renaissance a transitional period occurred, accompanied by a decline of feudalism and a rise in nationalism. With more vigorous trade and community growth, a stronger middle class gradually arose, with a resultant demand for an improved educational system designed to prepare the young male for his lifetime occupation. Some informal physical exercise and games contributed to the social and recreational goals of the young townspeople. Such physical activity also enhanced military training, and it is interesting to note that games and informal sports were accompanying features of the frequent religious holidays.

*The Renaissance.* The period that followed feudalism was known as the Renaissance. At this time it was natural that learned people should begin to look back to the periods in history that were characterized by even roughly similar societies. The Church was solidly entrenched, and there was much enthusiasm for scholarship in the fields of law, theology, and medicine. Understandably this scholasticism and emphasis on intellectual discipline found little if any room for physical education. Unorganized sports and games were the only activities of this nature in the cathedral schools and in the universities that had been established relatively recently. In the late 14th and in the 15th century, however, a type of humanism developed that stressed the worth of the individual--and once again the physical side of the person was considered. Most of the humanistic educators appreciated the earlier Greek ideal and emphasized the care and proper development of the body. Vittorino da Feltre set an example for others in his school at the court of the Prince of Mantua in northern Italy. One of his aims was to discipline the body so hardship might be endured with the least possible hazard. His pupils were some day to bear arms and had to know the art of warfare. Individual and group sports and games were included because of the recreational nature of such activity. Da Feltre believed that the ability of a youth to learn in the classroom depended to a considerable extent upon the physical condition of the individual, a belief for which there is some evidence today.

*Early Modern Period.* In what has been called the Early Modern Period, there followed a decline in liberal education as the schools lost their original aim and began the study of the languages of Greece and Rome exclusively while unfortunately neglecting the other aspects of these civilizations. The importance of physical training for youth again declined, even as preparation for life work was crowded out for many by preparation for university education. Thus, when the spirit of Italian humanistic education reached into Europe, the Greek ideal of athletics and physical education was realized by only a relatively few individuals. Those involved with the Protestant Reformation did practically nothing to encourage physical education activities with the possible exception of Martin Luther himself, who had an interest in wrestling  and who evidently realized a need for the physical training of youth. Some educators rebelled against the narrow type of education that came into vogue, but they were the exception rather than the rule.

For example, Rabelais satirized the education of the time in his depiction of the poor results of the typical Latin grammar school graduate. His Gargantua was a "dolt and blockhead," but subsequently became a worthwhile person when his education became more well- rounded. Also, Michel de Montaigne, the great French essayist of the 16th century, believed that the education of the person should not be dichotomized into the typical mind-body approach. Further, other educators such as Locke, Mulcaster, and Comenius recognized the value of physical exercise. Some educational leaders in the 17th century stressed character development as the primary educational aim, but a number of them believed in the underlying need for health and physical fitness. John Locke, for example, even stressed the importance of recreation for youth. However, his ideas were far from being accepted as the ideal for all in a society characterized by a variety of social classes.

*The 18th Century.* The 18th century in Europe was a period of change as to what might be called more modern political, social, and educational ideals. In France, Voltaire denounced both the Church and the state. Rousseau decried the state of society also, as well as the condition of education in this period. He appeared to desire equality for all and blamed the civilization of the time for the unhappiness in ther world (1943). He urged the adoption of a "back to nature" movement, because it seemed to him that everything had degenerated under the influence of what we have come to call organized society. In his heralded educational treatise *Emile*, he described what he considered to be the ideal education for a boy. From the age of 1 to 5, he stressed, the only concern should be for the growth and physical welfare of the young person. From 5 to twelve years of age, the idea of *natural* growth was to be continued as the strong, healthy youngster learned about the different aspects of his environment. Rousseau did consider the person to be an indivisible entity and was firmly convinced of the need to devote attention to the developmental growth of the *entire* organism. For him it was not possible to know when an activity lost its "physical" value and began to possess so-called "intellectual" worth.

At this point in Europe's history, many strong social forces, with the opinions of such men as Voltaire and Rousseau, led to the ruination of the existing political and social structure.  The reconstruction developed gradually in the 19th century concurrent with many changes, educational and otherwise, that influenced physical education  directly and indirectly. For example, Johann Basedow started a naturalistic school in Dessau based on the fundamental ideas of Rousseau. This school, called the Philanthropinum, was the first in modern Europe to admit children from all social classes and to give physical education a place in the daily curriculum. A number of other prominent educators during this period expressed what they felt to be the proper place of physical training in the curriculum. thereby helping to mold public opinion to a degree. Outstanding among these men were Guts Muths, Pestalozzi, and philosopher Immanuel Kant. Friedrich Froebel, who ranks along with Pestalozzi as a founder of modern pedagogy, offered the first planned program of education through play.

*Emerging Nationalism*. As it turned out, the rise of nationalism had a direct relationship to the development of physical education in modern Europe. Both the French and American revolutions sparked these feelings of strong loyalty to country in many parts of the world. Gradually, education was recognized as a vital means of promoting the progress of developing nations. Education for citizenship stressed the obligation of youth to develop itself fully for the glory of the nation. Historians have pointed out that nationalistic education is probably a necessary step toward subsequent internationalism, but it must be stated that still today it often brings grief to many in the process.

*Germany*. The Turnvereine (i.e., gymnastic societies) in Germany originated during the first decade of the 19th century. Freidrich L. Jahn, a staunch patriot of the time, is considered the father of this movement. He wished fervently that his people would become strong enough to throw off the yoke of the French conquerors. Jahn believed that exercise was a vital means to employ in the ideal plan of growth and development for the individual. He held also that there was a certain mental and moral training to be derived from experience at the Turnplatz (where exercises were performed). The War of Liberation for Prussia was waged successfully in 1813, and his work undoubtedly helped the cause. Turnen (German gymnastics) underwent periods of popularity and disfavor during the next 40 years. Later the Turnen societies accepted the games and sports of the sport movement cautiously.

Adolph Spiess did a great amount of work in planning and developing school gymnastics as he strove to have physical training included as an important part of the child's education. In 1849 he established normal classes in this type of gymnastics at Darmstadt. Since 1860 Germany has fully recognized the importance of school gymnastics, and this subject has continually grown in prominence for the pre-university years.

The military motive was very influential in shaping the development of physical training in a number of other European countries, with certain individual variations. Scientific advances have gradually brought about the inauguration of new theories in keeping with the advancing times.

*Great Britain.* Great Britain's isolated position in relation to the European continent made rigorous training for warfare and national defense less necessary and tended to foster the continuance of interest in outdoor sports. In feudal England archery was the most popular sport, and in the 15th century golf rivaled it until the king banned it by proclamation because of the disturbance it was creating. A bit later, however, it was accepted by nobles, and the ban was lifted. Field hockey, cricket, bowling, quoits, tennis, rugby, hammer throwing, and pole vaulting had their origins in the British Isles. Many of the other traditional sports originated elsewhere but were soon adopted by the people. In the early 19th century an urgent need was felt for some type of systematized physical training. Clias, Ehrenhoff, Georgii, and Maclaren were some of the men who introduced varied methods of physical training and culture to the British people. Any stress on systematized school gymnastics and the movement for improved health did not, however, discourage sport participation in any way. Down through years since then, Great Britain has encouraged active participation by all schoolchildren and avoided the overtraining of the few.

*The Modern Olympic Games.* The revival of the Olympic Games in 1896 was brought about largely through the efforts of Baron Pierre de Coubertin of France. Certainly much interest has been created with the successive holding of these Games every four years in countries all over the world. Although some are concerned about the media's preoccupation with team scores and the accompanying nationalistic flag-raising and the playing of national anthems, it probably can be argued successfully that international goodwill has been fostered by this highly competitive international sport. The cynic would counter by declaring that all of this "goodwill" resulted in two worldwide wars and innumerable sectional wars being fought since the advent of the modern Games. Assuredly, however, we must give some credence to the optimist's position that it has been worthwhile to promote such athletic competition in the hope that such "friendly strife" might have some constructive influence on the development of peace and international goodwill. Throughout the 20th century, therefore, sport and games for men, and then increasingly for women, too, became ever more popular throughout Europe and in most other parts of the world as well.

## Concluding Statement

There is obviously a value struggle going on that may well increase unless a continuing search for consensus is carried out. Such understanding at home and abroad will come only through greater understanding and wisdom applied in an atmosphere of international goodwill. Both science and philosophy will have to make their contributions. It is absolutely essential that there be careful study and analysis of the question of values as they relate to developmental physical activity in exercise, sport, and related expressive activities, a program that should be readily available to citizens of all ages and conditions across the world.

In a world with an uncertain future, there has been an ever-present demand for an improved level of physical fitness for citizens of all ages and conditions. The North American interest in all types of competitive sport has continued to grow unabated. Because of financial stringencies, overemphasis in certain areas, and deficiencies in others, unfortunately there is decreasing room for optimism.

# Chapter 6
## The Value Attached to Physical Activity (Including Sport) in American History

According to Norma Schwendener (1942), the history of physical education in the United America was divided into four distinct periods: (1) The Colonial Period (1609-1781); (2) The Provincial Period (1781-1885); (3) The Period of the Waning of European Influence (1885-1918); and (4) The Period of American Physical Education (1918- ). Although this classification will not be followed here, the reader can get some perspective from Schwendener's earlier outline.

### The Colonial Period

Living conditions in the American colonies in the 17th and 18th centuries were harsh, the finer elements of then civilized life being possible for only a relatively few wealthy individuals. The culture itself had been transported from Europe with its built-in class distinctions. The rules of primogeniture and entail served to strengthen such status. Slavery, and near-slavery, were general practice, especially in the South, and the right to vote was typically restricted to property owners. Cultural contrasts were marked. Religion was established legally. Geography, differences between the environment in the North and South, had a great deal to do with many differences that were evident. Actually, there was even considerable feeling against democratic principles both from a political and social standpoints. Any consideration of educational practice must, therefore, be viewed in the light of these conditions.1

Most of the American colonies established between 1607 and 1682 were guided in their educational outlook and activities by England's contemporary practices, the influence of other European countries being negligible at first. Education was thought to be a function of the Church, not the State. By today's standards, the provisions made for education were extremely inadequate. In a pioneer country characterized by a hazardous physical environment, the settlers were engaged in a daily struggle for their very existence. Early colonists migrated into different regions relatively close to the eastern coastline almost by chance. These differing environments undoubtedly influenced the social order of the North and the South; yet, for several generations there were many points of similarity in the traditions and experiences of the people as a whole. They all possessed a common desire for freedom and security, hopes that were to be realized only after a desperate struggle.

The church was the institution through which the religious heritage, and also much of the educational heritage, was preserved and advanced. The first schools can actually be regarded as the fruits of the Protestant revolts in Europe. The settlers wanted religious freedom, but the traditionalists among them insisted that a knowledge of the Gospel was required for personal salvation. The natural outcome was the creation of schools to help children learn to read; thus, it was the dominant Protestant churches that brought about the establishment of the elementary schools.

Three types of attitude developed toward education. The first was the compulsory-maintenance attitude of the New England Puritans, who established schools by colony legislation of 1642 and 1647. The second attitude was that of the parochial school, and this was best represented by Pennsylvania where private schools were made available for those who could afford it. The pauper-school, non-State-interference attitude was the third type. It was best exemplified by Virginia and the southern colonies. Many of these people had come to America for profit rather than religious freedom, the result being that they tended to continue school practice as it had existed in England. In all these schools, discipline was harsh and sometimes actually brutal. The curriculum consisted of the three R's and spelling, but the books were few and the teachers were generally unprepared.

The pattern of secondary education had been inherited from England too. In most of the colonies, and especially in New England, so-called Latin grammar schools appeared. Also, higher education was not neglected. Nine colleges were founded mainly through the philanthropy of special individuals or groups. In all of these institutions, theology formed an important part of the curriculum. A notable exception that began a bit later was the Academy and College of Philadelphia where Benjamin Franklin exerted a strong influence.

## Early Games, Contests, and Exercise

What about physical training and play for the young? What were the objectives for which people strove historically in what later was called physical education in the United States? We will now take a look at the different roles that such development physical activity played (or didn't play!) in the educational pattern of the States over a period of several centuries down to the present day. This entire time period covering the history of physical education in the United States could be divided logically into four distinct periods: the Colonial Period

(1609-1781); the Provincial Period (1781-1885); the Period of the Waning of European Influence (1885-1918); and the Period of American Physical Education (1918-   ).

Because the population of the colonial United States was mostly rural, one could not expect organized gymnastics and sports to find a place in the daily lives of the settlers. Most of the colonies, with the possible exception of the Puritans, engaged in the games and contests of their motherlands to the extent that they had free time. Even less than today, the significance of play and its possibilities in the educative process were not really comprehended; in fact, the entire educational system was opposed to the idea of what would be included in a fine program of sport and physical education today.

## The Eighteenth Century

With the advent of the 18th century, the former religious interest began to slacken. The government gradually developed more of a civil character with an accompanying tendency to create schools with a native vein or character. This was accompanied by a breakdown in some of the former aristocratic practices followed by a minority. The settled frontier expanded, new interests in trade and shipping grew, and the population increased. An evident trend toward individualism characterized this period as well. Several American industries date back to this time, the establishment of iron mills being most noteworthy.

Although the colonists were typically restricted by the financial practices placed by the English on the use of money, there was sufficient prosperity to bring about a change in the appearance of the established communities. An embryonic class structure began to form, with some colonials achieving a certain amount of social status by the holding of land and office. However, there were other concerns such as a series of small wars with the Spanish and the French extending from 1733 to 1763. These struggles were interspersed by period of cold war maneuvering. What was called the Seven Years' War (1755-1763) ended with the colonies as a fairly solid political and economic unit. However, the British method of governance over the colony was a constant source of annoyance and serious concern with the result that a strong nationalistic, separatist feeling emerging about 1775.

Beginning in the third decade of the eighteenth century, a revival of religious interest was apparent. This occasioned a recurring strong emphasis on religious education in the elementary schools. However, with the stirring of economic, political, and nationalistic forces from approximately 1750 onward, a period of relative religious tolerance resulted. This was accompanied by a broader interest in national affairs by many. The result was a lesser emphasis on the earlier religious domination of the elementary curriculum.

Secondary education was still provided by the grammar schools. These schools, generally located in every large town, were supported by the local government and by private tuition. The curricula were non-utilitarian and were designed to prepare boys for college entrance. Insofar as higher education was concerned, the pattern had been established from the beginning (Harvard College in 1636) after the European university type of liberal arts education with a strong emphasis on mental discipline and theology.

Despite the above, the reader should keep in mind that there were still very few heavily populated centers. In the main, frontier life especially, but also life in small villages, was still most rigorous. Such conditions were simply not conducive to intellectual life with high educational standards. Educational theorists had visions of a fine educational system, of course, but state constitutional provisions regarding education were very limited, and the federal constitution didn't say anything about educational standards at all. The many new social forces at work offered some promise, but with the outbreak of the War of Independence formal education came to almost a complete standstill.

The last twenty-fice years of the 18th century saw a great many changes in the life of the United States. In the first place, many of the revolutionaries who started the war lived to tell about it and to help in the sound reconstruction of the young nation. State and federal constitutions had to be planned, written, and approved. Also, it was very important to the early success of the country that commerce be revived, a process that was accomplished sooner by the South because of the nature of the commodities they produced. New lines of business and trade were established with Russia, Sweden, and the Orient. The Federal Convention of 1787 managed to complete what has turned out to be possibly the most successful document in all of history, the Constitution of the United States of America. Then George Washington's administration began, and it was considered successful both at home and abroad. Interestingly, the concurrent French Revolution became an issue in American politics, but Washington persuaded his government to declare a position of neutrality (although he was hard pressed to maintain it).

As soon as the War of Independence in the U.S. was over, considerable attention was turned to education with the result that higher and secondary education improved. The colleges of the North took longer to recover from the War than those in the South where soon an imposing list of both private, religiously endowed, and state-sponsored institutions were founded.

## Early Support for Physical Training

At the secondary level, the institutions that succeeded the Latin grammar schools became known as the academies. Their aim was to prepare youth to meet life and its many problems, a reflection of the main influences of the Enlightenment in America. With such an emphasis, it is natural that the physical welfare of youths gradually was considered to be more important that it had been previously. Some of the early academies, such as Dummer, Andover, Exeter, and Leicester, were founded and incorporated before 1790. This movement reached its height around 1830 when there was said to be approximately 800 such schools throughout the country.

Many of the early American educators and statesmen supported the idea that both the body and the mind needed attention in our educational system. Included among this number were Benjamin Franklin, Noah Webster, Thomas Jefferson, Horace Mann, and Henry Barnard. Further support came from Captain Alden Partridge, one of the early superintendents of the United States Military Academy at West Point, who crusaded for the reform of institutions of higher education. He deplored the entire neglect of physical culture.

## The Nineteenth Century

With the stage set for the United States to enter a most important period in her history, the 19th century witnessed steady growth along with a marked increase in nationalism. There was a second war with Great Britain, the War of 1812. In the ensuing nationalist era, many political changes or "adjustments" were carried out in relations with Britain and other nations where necessary. The Monroe Doctrine declared to the world that countries in this hemisphere should be left alone to develop as they saw fit and were not to be used by outside powers for colonization. However, at home dissent was growing as the North and the South were being divided. The North was being changed by virtue of the Industrial Revolution taking place, along with many educational and humanitarian movements. The South, conversely, continued to nurture a different type of society regulated by what has been called a slave and cotton economy.

In the realm of education, the first 50 years of the new national life was a period of transition from the control of the church to that of the State. State control and support gradually seemed more feasible, although the change was seemingly slow in coming. The desire for political equality and religious freedom, along with changing economic conditions, finally made education for all a necessity. By 1825, therefore, a tremendous struggle for the creation of the American State School was underway. In the field of public education, the years from 1830 to 1860 have been regarded by some educational historians as "The Architectural Period."

North American Turners. In the early 19th century German gymnastics (*Turnen*) came to the United States through the influx of such men as Charles Beck, Charles Follen, and Francis Lieber. However, the majority of the people were simply not ready to recognize the possible values of these activities imported from foreign lands. The Turnverein movement (in the late 1840s) before the Civil War was very important for the advancement of physical training. The Turners advocated that mental and physical education should proceed hand in hand in the public schools. As it developed, they were the leaders in the early physical education movement around 1850 in such cities as Boston, St. Louis, and Cincinnati.

Other leaders in this period were George Barker Win(d)ship and Dioclesian Lewis. Windship was an advocate of heavy gymnastics and did much to convey the mistaken idea that great strength should be the goal of all gymnastics, as well as the notion that strength and health were completely synonymous. Lewis, who actually began the first teacher training program in physical education in the country in 1861, was a crusader in every sense of the word; he had ambitions to improve the health of all Americans through his system of light calisthenics--an approach that he felt would develop and maintain flexibility, grace, and agility as well. His stirring addresses to many professional and lay groups did much to popularize this type of gymnastics, and to convey the idea that such exercise could serve a desirable role in the lives of those who were weaker and perhaps even sickly (as well as those who were naturally stronger).

The Civil War between the North and the South wrought a tremendous change in the lives of the people. In the field of education, the idea of equality of educational opportunity had made great strides; the "educational ladder" was gradually extending upward with increasing opportunity for even more young people. For example, the number of high schools increased fivefold between 1870 and 1890. The state was gradually assuming a position of prime importance in public education. In this process, state universities were helpful as they turned their attention to advancing the welfare of the individual states. The Southern states lagged behind the rest of the country due to the ravages of War with subsequent reconstruction, racial conflict, and continuing fairly "aristocratic theory" of education. In the North, however, President Eliot of Harvard called for education reform in 1888. One of his main points was the need for greatly improved teacher training.

After the Civil War, the Turners through their societies continued to stress the benefits of physical education within public education. Through their efforts it was possible to reach literally hundreds of thousands of people either directly or indirectly. The Turners have always opposed military training as a substitute for physical education. Further, the modern playground movement found the Turners among its strongest supporters. The Civil War had demonstrated clearly the need for a concerted effort in the areas of health, physical education, and physical recreation (not to mention competitive sports and games). The Morrill Act passed by Congress in 1862 helped create the land-grant colleges. At first, the field of physical education was not aided significantly by this development because of the stress on military drill in these institutions. All in all, the best that can be said is that an extremely differentiated pattern of physical education was present in the post-Civil War of the country.

## Beginning of Organized Sport in America

The beginning of organized sport in America, as we now know it, dates back approximately to the Civil War period. Baseball and tennis were introduced in that order during this period and soon became very popular. Golf, bowling, swimming, basketball, and a multitude of other so-called minor sports made their appearance in the latter half of the nineteenth century. American football also started its rise to popularity at this time. The Amateur Athletic Union was organized in 1888 to provide governance for amateur sport. Unfortunately, controversy about amateurism has surrounded this organization almost constantly ever since. Nevertheless, it has given invaluable service to the promotion of that changing and often evanescent phenomenon that this group has designated as "legitimate amateur sport."

## The Young Men's Christian Association'

The YMCA traces its origins back to 1844 in London, England, when George Williams organized the first religious group. This organization has always stressed as one of its basic principles that physical welfare and recreation were helpful to the moral wellbeing of the individual. Some of the early outstanding physical education leaders in the YMCA in the United States were Robert J. Roberts, Luther Halsey Gulick, and James Huff McCurdy.

## Early Physical Activity at the College Level

It was toward the middle of the 19th century that the colleges and universities began to think seriously about the health of their students. The University of Virginia had the first real gymnasium, and Amherst College followed in 1860 with a two-story structure devoted to physical education. President Stearns urged the governing body to begin a department of physical culture in which the primary aim was to keep the student in good physical condition. Dr. Edward Hitchcock headed this department for an unprecedented period of fifty years until his death in 1911. Yale and Harvard erected gymnasiums for similar purposes in the late 1800s, but their programs were not supported adequately until the early 1900s. These early facilities were soon followed elsewhere by the development of a variety of "exercise buildings" built along similar lines.

Harvard was fortunate in the appointment of Dr. Dudley Allen Sargent to Hemenway Gymnasium. This dedicated physical educator and physician led the university to a preeminent position in the field, and his program became a model for many other colleges and universities. He stressed physical education for the individual. His goal was the attainment of a perfect structure--harmony in a well-balanced development of mind and body.

From the outset, college faculties had taken the position that games and sports were not necessarily a part of the basic educational program. Interest in them was so intense, however, that the wishes of the students, while being denied, could not be thwarted. Young college men evidently strongly desired to demonstrate their abilities in the various sports against presumed rivals from other institutions. Thus, from 1850 to 1880 the rise of interest in intercollegiate sports was phenomenal. Rowing, baseball, track and field, football, and later basketball were the major sports. Unfortunately, college representatives soon found that the athletic sports needed control as evils began to creep in and partially destroy the values originally intended as goals.

## An Important Decade for Physical Education

The years from 1880 to 1890 undoubtedly form one of the most important decades in the history of physical education in the United States. The colleges and universities, the YMCAs, the Turners, and the proponents of the various foreign systems of gymnastics made contributions during this brief period. The Association for the Advancement of Physical Education (now AAHPERD) was founded in 1885, with the word "American" being added the next year. This professional organization was the first of its kind in the field and undoubtedly stimulated teacher education markedly. An important early project was the plan for developing a series of experiences in physical activity--physical education--the objectives of which would be in accord with the existing pattern of general education. The struggle to bring about widespread adoption of such a program followed. Early legislation implementing physical education was enacted in five states before the turn of the 20th century.

The late 19th century saw the development also of the first efforts in organized recreation and camping for children living in underdeveloped areas in large cities. The first playground was begun in Boston in 1885. New York and Chicago followed suit shortly thereafter, no doubt to a certain degree as a result of the ill effects of the Industrial Revolution. This was actually the meager beginning of the present tremendous recreation movement in our country. Camping, both that begun by private individuals and organizational camping, started before the turn of the century as well; it has flourished similarly since that time and has been an important supplement to the entire movement.

Although criticism of the educational system as a whole was present between 1870 and 1890, it really assumed large scale proportions in the last decade of the 19th century. All sorts of innovations and reforms were being recommended from a variety of quarters. The social movement in education undoubtedly had a relationship to a rise in political progressivism. Even in the universities, the formalism present in psychology, philosophy, and the social sciences was coming under severe attack. Out in the public schools, a different sort of conflict was raging. Citizens were demanding that the promise of American life should be reflected through change and a broadening of the school's purposes. However, although the seeds of this educational revolution were sown in the 19th century, the story of its accomplishment belongs to the present century.

## The Twentieth Century

The tempo of life in America seemed to increase in the 20th century. The times were indeed changing as evidenced, for example, by one war after another. In retrospect there were so many wars--World War I, World War II, the Korean War, the Vietnam War, and the seemingly ever-present "cold war" after the global conflict of the 1940s. They inescapably had a powerful influence of society along with the worldwide depression of the 1930s. Looking back on 20th century history is frightening; so much has happened, and it has happened so quickly. The phenomenon of change is as ubiquitous today as are the historic nemeses of death and taxes.

In the public realm, social legislation and political reform made truly significant changes in the lives of people despite the leavening, ever-present struggle between conservative and liberal forces. Industry and business assumed gigantic proportions, as did the regulatory controls of the federal government. The greatest experiment in political democracy in the history of the world was grinding ahead with deliberate speed, but with occasional stopping-off sessions while "breath was caught." The idealism behind such a plan that amounted to "democratic socialism" was at times being challenged from all quarters. Also, wars and financial booms and depressions (or later recessions) weren't the types of developments that made planning and execution simple matters. All of these developments mentioned above have had their influence on the subject at hand--education (and, of course, physical education and sport).

In the early 20th century, United States citizens began to do some serious thinking about their educational aims or values. The earliest aim in U.S. educational history had been religious in nature, an approach that was eventually supplanted by a political aim consistent with emerging nationalism. But then an overwhelming utilitarian, economic aim seemed to overshadow the political aim. The tremendous increase in high school enrollment forced a reconsideration of the aims of education at all levels of the system. Training for the elite was supplanted by an educational program to be mastered by the many. It was at this time also that the beginnings of a scientific approach to educational problems forced educators to take stock of the development based on theory and a scholarly rationale other than one forced on the school simply because of a sheer increase in numbers.

Then there followed an effort on the part of many people to consider aims and objectives from a sociological orientation. For the first time, education was conceived in terms of complete living as a citizen of an evolving democracy. The influence of John Dewey and others encouraged the viewing of the curriculum as child-centered rather than subject-centered--a rather startling attempt to alter the long-standing basic orientation that involved the rote mastery of an amalgam of educational source material. The Progressive Education Movement placed great emphasis on individualistic aims. This was subsequently countered by a demand for a theory stressing a social welfare orientation rather than one so heavily pointed to individual development.

The relationship between health education and physical education grew extensively during the first quarter of the 20th century, and this included their liaison with the entire system of education. Health education in all its aspects was viewed seriously, especially after the evidence surfaced from the draft statistics of World War I. Many states passed legislation requiring varying amounts of time in the curriculum devoted to the teaching of physical education. National interest in sports and games grew at a phenomenal rate in an era when economic prosperity prevailed. The basis for school and community recreation was being well-laid.

Simultaneously with physical education's achievement of a type of maturity brought about legislation designed to promote physical fitness and healthy bodies, the struggle between the inflexibility of the various foreign systems of gymnastics and the individual freedom of the so-called "natural movement" was being waged with increasing vigor. Actually the rising interest in sports and games soon made the conflict unequal, especially when the concept of "athletics for all" really began to take hold in the second and third decades of the century.

**Conflicting Educational Philosophies**

Even today the significance of play and its possibilities in the educative process have not really been comprehended. In fact, until well up in the 1800s in America, the entire educational system was opposed to the entire idea of what would be included in a fine program of sport and physical education today. It was the organized German-American Turners primarily, among certain others, who came to this continent from their native Germany and advocated that mental and physical education should proceed hand in hand in the public schools. The Turners' opposition to military training as a substitute for physical education contributed to the extremely differentiated pattern of physical education in the post-Civil War era. Their influence offset the stress on military drill in the land-grant colleges created by Congress passing the Morrill Act in the United States in 1862. The beginning of U.S. sport as we know it also dates to this period and, from the outset, college faculties took the position that games and sport were not a part of the basic educational program. The colleges and universities, the YMCAs, the Turners, and the proponents of the various foreign systems of gymnastics made significant contributions during the last quarter of the 19th century.

In the early 20th century Americans began to do some earnest thinking about their educational aims and values. Whereas the earliest aim in U.S. educational history had been religious in nature, this was eventually supplanted by a political aim consistent with emerging nationalism. But then an overwhelming utilitarian, economic aim seemed to overshadow the political aim. It was at this time also that the beginnings of a scientific approach to educational problems forced educators to take stock of the development based on a rationale other than the sheer increase in student enrollment.

Then there followed an effort to consider aims and objectives from a sociological orientation. For the first time, education was conceived in terms of complete living as a citizen in an evolving democracy. The influence of John Dewey and others encouraged the viewing of the curriculum as child-centered rather than subject-centered. Great emphasis was placed on individualistic aims with a subsequent counter demand for a theory stressing more of a social welfare orientation.

The relationship between health and physical education and the entire system of education strengthened during the first quarter of the 20th century. Many states passed legislation requiring physical education in the curriculum, especially after the damning evidence of the draft statistics in World War I (Van Dalen, Bennett, and Mitchell, 1953, p. 432). Simultaneous with physical education's achievement of a type of maturity through such legislation, the struggle between the inflexibility of the various foreign systems of gymnastics and the individualistic freedom of the so-called "natural movement" was being waged with increasing vigor. Actually the rising interest in sports and games soon made the conflict unequal, especially when the concept of athletics for all really began to take hold in the second and third decades of the century.

The natural movement was undoubtedly strengthened further by much of the evidence gathered by many natural and social scientists. A certain amount of the spirit of Dewey's philosophy took hold within the educational environment, and this new philosophy and accompanying methodology and techniques did appear to be more effective in the light of the changing ideals of an evolving democracy. Despite this pragmatic influence, however, the influence of idealism remained

103

strong also, with its emphasis on the development of individual personality and the possible inculcation of moral and spiritual values through the transfer of training theory applied to sports and games.

**Embryonic Emergence of the "Allied Professions"**

School health education was developed greatly during the period also. The scope of school hygiene increased, and a required medical examination for all became more important. Leaders were urged to conceive of school health education as including three major divisions: health services, health instruction, and healthful school living. The value of such expansion in this area was gradually accepted by educator and citizen alike. For example, many physical educators began to show a concern for a broadening of the field's aims and objectives, the evidence of which could be seen by the increasing amount of time spent by many on coaching duties. Conversely, the expansion of health instruction through the medium of many public and private agencies tended to draw those more directly interested in the goals of health education away from physical education.

Progress in the recreation field was significant as well. The values inherent in well-conducted playground activities for children and youths were increasingly recognized; the Playground Association of America was organized in 1906. At this time there was still an extremely close relationship between physical education and recreation, a link that remained strong because of the keen interest in the aims of recreation by a number of outstanding physical educators. Many municipal recreation centers were constructed, and it was at this time that the use of some-- relatively few, actually--of the schools for "after-hour" recreation began. People began to recognize that recreational activities served an important purpose in a society undergoing basic changes. Some recreation programs developed under local boards of education; others were formed by the joint sponsorship of school boards and municipal governments; and a large number of communities placed recreation under the direct control of the municipal government and either rented school facilities when possible, or gradually developed recreational facilities of their own.

**The Various Professional Associations
Form an Alliance**

The American Association for Health, Physical Education, and Recreation (now the American Alliance for Health, Physical Education, Recreation, and Dance) has accomplished a great deal in a strong united effort to coordinate the various allied professions largely within the framework of public and private education. Despite membership losses during the 1970s, its success story continues with those functions which properly belong within the educational sphere. The Alliance should in time also gradually increase its influence on those seeking those services and opportunities that we can provide at the various other age levels as well.

Of course, for better or worse, there are many other health agencies and groups, recreational associations and enterprises, physical education associations and "splinter" disciplinary groups, and athletics associations and organizations moving in a variety of directions. One example of these is the North American Society for Sport Management that began in the mid-1980s and has grown significantly since. Each of these is presumably functioning with the system of values and norms prevailing in the country (or culture, etc.) and the resultant pluralistic educational philosophies extant within such a milieu.

We have seen teacher education generally, under which physical education has been bracketed, and professional preparation for recreational leadership also, strengthened through self-evaluation and accreditation. The dance movement has been a significant development within the educational field, and those concerned are still determining the place for this movement within the educational program at all levels. A great deal of progress has been made in physical education, sport, and (more recently) kinesiology research since 1960.

## Achieving Some Historical Perspective

It is now possible to achieve some historical perspective about the second and third quarters of the 20th century as they have affected physical education and sport, as well as the allied professions of health education, recreation, and dance education. The Depression of the 1930s, World War II, the Korean War, and then Vietnam War, and the subsequent cold war with the many frictions among countries have been strong social forces directly influencing sport, physical education, health education, recreation, and dance in any form and in any country. Conversely, to what extent these various fields and their professional concerns have in turn influenced the many cultures, societies, and social systems remains yet to be accurately determined.

It would be simplistic to say that physical educators want more and better physical education and intramural recreational sport programs, that athletics oriented coaches and administrators want more and better athletic competition, that health and safety educators want more and better health and safety education, that recreation personnel want more and better recreation, and that dance educators want more and better dance instruction--and yet, this would probably be a correct assessment of their wishes and probably represents what has occurred to a large degree.

## Specialization in American Professional Preparation in Physical Education Teaching/Coaching and Disciplinary Study in Kinesiology

In 1988, Zeigler (pp. 177-196) reported the results of a comparative investigation of the undergraduate professional preparation programs in physical education in the United States and Canada based on his own investigation of both the theoretical and the practical aspects of training programs in both countries. Hypothesizing that there have been significant changes, some similar and others in markedly different directions in the past quarter century (from approximately 1960 to 1985), he further hypothesized that, if and when changes did occur, they tended to come about in the United States first. This latter hypothesis was based on the author's personal experience in both countries, and also on the results of a study by Lipset (1973). Lipset had pointed out that there has been reluctance on the part of Canadians "to be overly optimistic, assertive, or experimentally inclined." Based on the results of this investigation, however, such has not necessarily been the case in the field of physical education and sport (see also Zeigler, 1980).

To report more accurately on this subject for the 1980s, and also to gain a better perspective on the the United States' scene, seven members of the American Academy of Physical Education, distributed geographically across the country, each who have been involved in professional preparation for periods up to 40 years, were asked to describe what they believe took place in the United States over three different time periods (i.e., during the 1960s, the 1970s, and the 1980s). What follows here, then, is delimited to their responses for the period covering the 1980s and also to the investigation and analysis carried out personally by the author.

Five problems, phrased as questions, were included in the questionnaire as follows: (1) what have been the strongest social influences during the current decade? (2) what changes have been made in the professional curriculum? (3) what developments have taken place in instructional methodology? (4) what other interesting or significant developments have occurred (typically within higher education)? (5) what are the greatest problems in professional preparation currently?

## Strongest Social Influences

During the 1980s, a number of strong social influences were indicated on the United States scene. Worldwide communication was improving greatly as ever more satellites were put into service. Nevertheless, the seemingly ever-present concern with the several violently conflicting world ideologies remained at a high level of intensity as the decade began. The Reagan administration displayed an aggressive "proud to be American" leadership style, along with emphasis on strong offensive and defensive military concerns, in an ongoing struggle to combat spreading communism at numerous points around the globe. Others were worried that the United States was overextending itself through "imperial overstretch" in its zeal to make the world safe for democracy (Kennedy, 1987, p. 515).

A variety of new and continuing problems and issues were apparent on the home front as well, some having both positive and negative implications for the future. The impact of high technology (e.g., computers, software--the entire "knowledge industry" for that matter) was felt increasingly. Certain large industries were suffering greatly from cheaper foreign competition (e.g., steel production), but fortunately the North American car market held up (to some extent through wise partial mergers with foreign competitors).

The cost of education soared at all educational levels, while concurrently funding from the federal level was decreasing. Greater cooperation between the public schools and higher educational institutions was apparent. With an enrollment decline beginning to have an effect on many colleges and universities, there was increased competition for top students. A presidential task force on the state of education was proclaiming a "prevalence of mediocrity" in the secondary schools. This demand for accountability at a very high level brought about a steady call throughout the decade for a "back to basics" movement in education. It was argued that "teachers can't teach," but others were promoting the idea of "mastery teaching" (an idea that makes sense upon first examination). However, some wanted students promoted anyhow because age differentials were creating more disciplinary problems. Developments that impacted on physical education were (1) the federal government easing off on Title IX enforcement that took some pressure off state legislatures to provide equal opportunity for girls and women in sport, and (2) there was evidence that less than one third of the total school population (ages 10-17) received daily physical education.

## The Physical Education/Kinesiology Curriculum

Along with the continued expansion of non-teaching options or areas of concentration within the physical education-kinesiology major program (s), there was a concurrent decline of interest in under–girding liberal education and an evident increase in the importance of job orientation. Many felt there was a need to eliminate what they regarded as superfluous courses, while stressing the need for improved scholarship within those that remained.  The feeling was that students were typically more serious and goal-oriented, but the concern and pressure for high numerical grades was disconcerting to some observers.

Interestingly, and unfortunately, there has been an increased number of students with relatively poor physical skills in the professional/disciplinary programs.  Whether this trend was counteracted by an improvement in theoretical understanding remain debatable, however.  In the final analysis, however, it should be recognized that each university can't be "all things to all people" with its program offerings.

The 1980s witnessed also a new emphasis on special physical education because of state legislation, but such specialization within professional preparation programs was still not sufficiently available. There was also continued concern, but not much concrete action, for improved standards as evidenced by state certification for alternate career graduates and/or voluntary national accreditation for such programs related to ongoing teacher education programs.  One promising note was the establishment of a National Association for Sport and Physical Education (NASPE) Task Force working on a revision of accreditation standards for undergraduate physical education teacher preparation.

Along with declining enrollment in professional curricula, there was a need to generate increased revenue. Faculty positions were being lost due to inadequate funding, and intra-institutional research funding was drying up.

## Instructional Methodology

Several definite observations can be safely made in connection with instructional methodology. The weakening financial situation brought about a collapsing of course sections into larger lecture groups. This created a problem, however, because there was also been continued concern for teacher/coach effectiveness. Many faculty members began to take their teaching responsibilities more seriously, and there appeared to be an improved level of innovation and creativity in their efforts. This trend was accompanied by the retooling of certain faculty members to improve their instructional competency, thereby making them more valuable to their faculty units. There is no doubt but that course content has been based somewhat more on research findings and improved theory. Computer instruction is gradually being incorporated into the instructional pattern in a variety of ways, as is increased use of videotaping. The need to somehow streamline the learning experiences was expressed, as was a concern that there be greater stress on education for "human fulfillment" with the teacher as facilitator.

## Other Campus Developments

At the beginning of the 1980s, the continuing, bleak financial picture brought about a considerable degree of faculty pessimism and cynicism. Requirements for promotion and tenure were ever more stringent, while at the same time faculty positions were threatened because of continued economic pressures. Salary schedules did not keep pace with many other professions and occupations.

Sub-disciplinary specialization of faculty members increased steadily in the larger universities. With such broadly based (i.e., research and publication, heavier teaching/coaching workloads), the prevailing dictum seemed to be: Get the research grant no matter whether there is time to complete the project. Early retirement schemes appeared, but they were often not sufficiently creative or rewarding to encourage faculty departure. All in all, there was the feeling that the environment was too stressful.

## The Greatest Problems or Needs
## In Professional Preparation
## And Discipline Specialization

As the 20th century was drawing to a close, a number of problems expressed as needs were identified as follows:

1. Need to develop consensus about a disciplinary definition from which should evolve a more unified, much less fractionated curriculum (i.e., a greater balance among the bio-scientific aspects, the social-science & humanities aspects, and the "professional aspects" of our field).

2. Need to develop a sound body of retrievable knowledge in all phases of the profession's work.

3. Need to implement the educational possibilities of a competency approach within the professional preparation curriculum.
4. Need to develop a variety of sound options for specialization within a unified curriculum (extending to a 5th year of offerings?). This involves the expansion of alternate career options in keeping with the profession's goal of serving people of all ages and all abilities.
5. Need to develop a format whereby regular future planning between staff and students occurs.
6. Need to graduate competent, well-educated, fully professional physical educator/coaches who have sound personal philosophies embodying an understanding of professional ethics.
7. Need to seek recognition of our "professional endeavors" in public, semi-public, and private agency work through certification at the state level and voluntary accreditation at the national level.
8. Need to help control or lessen the impact of highly competitive athletics within the college and university structure so that a finer type of professional preparation program is fostered.
9. Need to recognize the worth of intramural recreational sports in our programs, and to make every effort to encourage those administering these programs to maintain "professional" identification with the National Association for Sport and Physical Education and the American Association for Physical Activity and Recreation.
10. Need to continue the implementation of patterns of administrative control in educational institutions that are fully consonant with individual freedom within the society.
11. Need to work for maintenance of collegiality among faculty members despite the inroads of factors that are tending to destroy such a

state: lack of adequate funding, faculty
unionization, pressure for publication and the
obtaining of grants, and extensive
intra-profession splintering.

12. Need to develop an attitude that will permit
us to "let go of obsolescence." Somehow we
will have to learn to apply new knowledge
creatively in the face of an often discouraging
political environment.

13. Need to work to dispel any malaise present
within our professional preparation programs
in regard to the future of the field.
If we prepare our students to be certified and
accredited professionals in their respective
options within the broad curriculum, we will
undoubtedly bring about a service profession
of the highest type within a reasonable period
of time.

## Concluding Statement

As these words are being written, there is obviously a continuing value
struggle going on in the United States that results in distinct swings of the
educational pendulum to and fro. It seems most important that a continuing search
for a consensus be carried out. Fortunately, the theoretical struggle fades a bit
when actual educational practice is carried out. If this were not so, very little
progress would be possible. If we continue to strive for improved educational
standards for all this should result in the foreseeable future in greater
understanding and wisdom on the part of the majority of North American citizens.
In this regard science and philosophy can and indeed must make ever-greater
contributions. All concerned members of the allied fields in both the United States
and Canada need to be fully informed as they strive for a voice in shaping the
future development of their respective countries and professions. It is essential that
there be careful and continuing study and analysis of the question of values as they
relate to sport, exercise, dance, and play. Such study and analysis is, of course,
basic as well to the implications that societal values and norms have for the allied
fields of physical (activity) education, health & safety education, recreation, dance,
and sport management.

Note: The information about the United States has been adapted from several sources, sections or parts of reports or books written earlier by the author. See Zeigler, 1951, 1962, 1975, 1979, 1988a, 1988b, 1990, 2003, 2005.

# Chapter 7
# The Evolving Value Orientation
# of
# Physical Activity Education
# in Twentieth–Century America

This chapter opens with a two-part general question that requires an answer as North America looks to the future. The question is: *How did it happen historically that the public educational system in North America has ended up with (1) a universal "varsity" sport program for the gifted and (2) a typically inadequate or non-existent physical activity education and intramural-sport program for the large majority of normal and special-needs children, youth, and young adults?*

I originally thought it would be possible to separate my overall treatment about the development of physical education and sport into two questions with appropriate chapters or parts. First I would relate what happened to sport in North American in the twentieth century. Then I would follow this with a *second* chapter explaining what needed to happen to rectify what I consider turned into an unsatisfactory situation.

My plan was to also have a *third* chapter describing what happened in the development of (what I now call) physical activity education during the past century. A *fourth* chapter to follow that immediately *with another section* in which I would offer recommendations about what *should* happen to physical activity education in the 21st century to rectify to be what I consider the present unsatisfactory, inadequate situation throughout America (and one that extends to an unknown degree in Canada).

My original plan soon went awry because it simply was not possible to separate the two (i.e., physical education and sport) in that manner. This is so because early in the twentieth century the physical education profession incorporated the teaching of sport skills in its curriculum. At the same time "sport professionals" were proceeding merrily on their way blithely uninterested and unconcerned with a concept of "physical activity education with related, appropriate health education" for all.

## The Turning Point in American Physical Education

Hence, in my efforts at historical scholarship about the North American scene (America and Canada), I found myself challenged to explain fully and correctly how this "tale of woe came to be" as North American society developed. Then I recalled VanderZwaag's analysis about what occurred during the period from 1880-1920 in the United States (1975). He explained that "the nineteenth century was characterized by sectional interests and struggles among systems in physical education. This would not seem to be true today. We have a "system," but what is it? What was the turning point after which "something" has emerged that we might identify as an American (or North American) system of "physical (activity) education (including sport and related health instruction)"?

VanderZwaag explained an answer to the emergence of "something" in the early twentieth century. The answer was to be found in:

> the steadily increasing interest in sports among the American people. The popularity of athletic contests was evident long before 1880. However, the earliest interest was developed through athletic clubs and intercollegiate athletics. The mass of the people did not receive the educational benefits to be derived from such activity.

As it turned out, it could be argued that a perverted British sporting pattern of "extra-curricular sport" won out over the several foreign systems of physical education. As VanderZwaag explained further, by 1920 it was evident that the United States had evolved a program of physical education that was characterized by informality and emphasis upon national sports. Such a program was thought to be entirely natural in view of our changing educational and political philosophies.

Educationally, there was a growing recognition that a sound program of education should be based upon the needs of the child. This was also being recognized in the field of physical education that rapidly came to a system of physical education for the public schools that was based upon the play activities of childhood. However, the reader may ask immediately: "Why did this acceptance of "play and sport" as "physical education" materialize? Seeking to answer this question more fully, I remembered that many years ago. When I was thesis adviser to the late Phyllis J. Hill at the University of Illinois, UIUC, she provided an explanation in her investigation completed in 1965 (*A Cultural History of Sport in Illinois, 1673-1820).* In her concluding statement, she wrote: "I am forced to the position that American cultural practices, including sport, have been forged by environmental forces, rather than by Anglo-Saxon tradition". This conclusion has merit still today because as she explained further, "work ethics and sport ethics are so close as to be virtually indistinguishable."

I sought to comprehend more completely what this means for us *today* in the field of physical (activity) education and (educational) sport. Hill had concluded: "if all human behavior is, indeed, a total and patterned response, *the understanding of sport can be furthered only when it is studied in reference to other human variables within the culture*" [the emphasis is by EFZ].

## The Original Ideal Was Perverted

What can I conclude today? I can only affirm that the original goal of early physical education professionals in the late 1800s was sound educationally. However, other societal influences were brought to bear on the ideal thereby perverting it. Today many in the profession believe that our task is still physical activity education, including educational–recreational sport and related health instruction, *designed to help all youth of all ages and conditions (!)* understand how important it is for them to be involved in a type of developmental physical activity that will enable them to *live life more fully* based on their choice of "life values." If they choose correctly, and we in the field help them acquire the needed knowledge and skills to live life more fully, the evidence we have from research now points to *a longer life for them as well* for those who choose wisely…

However, I believe that a wise, concerned person today can only be discouraged about the inexorable "decline" of what I would call "ideal" competitive sport in the 20th century. I am not talking about the current drug issue, actually a significant, horrendous problem, but about the rampant commercialism extending far and wide as I write these words. For example, most recently flag football for girls has been well received in Florida and seems ideal for competitive purposes. Nevertheless, parents are already complaining that daughters participating in this non-gate receipt sport won't have a chance for college scholarships!

Perhaps I should just "shut up" on the subject of developments in the sport realm. However, I am sad to say that the "higher realm" of sport has simply not evolved as I hoped it would. Many of you will get to see what happens down the line, but not me at age 92. I can still hope, however, that sensible people "out there" will somehow be able to lessen the impact of the commercial forces in sport to a reasonable extent. I—and like-minded people of my generation—just could not seem to manage it.

I recall that, as a youngster in New York City in the 1920s, I rooted for the Yankees and such players as Lou Gehrig and Babe Ruth (more for the former because he was also a wonderful person in so many respects). I played high school and college sport in New England in the 1930s, when sport was kept more in perspective with life's other aspects. Subsequently, in the 1940s and 1950s, I coached three sports (football and swimming or wrestling alternately) at Yale and Western Ontario. It was still "educational" and "recreational" then, too. When I moved to Michigan (Ann Arbor) in the late 1950s and early 1960s, however, I began to see that–even in that great university–the "tail was wagging the dog" too frequently. One professor went on all away football trips and was known as the "a-b-c lady" (i.e., she typically awarded "A's" for athletes, "B's" for boys, and "C's" for coeds unless the latter were outstanding students and she obviously had to grade them higher.

However, it was at Illinois (Urbana-Champaign), as department head of physical education in the 1960s, that I first encountered the cheating and under-the-table chicanery of a relatively small number of my own faculty members (coaches). And, sadly, I found I was powerless–even as the department head–to learn the facts of the matter, much less have anything to say or do about it. The president's office took over when football and basketball "problems" erupted and became the "Illinois Slush-Fund Scandal" in 1966-67 in the Big Ten Conference. So I decided to get out of administration fast. If a department head cannot even find out what his faculty members are being charged with—what the hell!

Fortunately I was able to "retreat" to Canada in 1971 as dean of a new faculty (college) at The University of Western Ontario. There—for the second time—I found that I had authentic student-athletes in class. The first term back I did not even know who were the varsity football and basketball athletes in my classes. (In addition, no coaches were calling me weekly to check on whether their "hot dogs" were attending classes.) This made me feel "whole" again regarding the relationship of physical activity education and intercollegiate athletics within education.

**Highly Competitive Sport's Worth to Society?**

So, what can I say to competitive sport in the United States–either with educational circles or in society at large–as I gradually but steadily fade from the picture? I can only ask, "Is highly competitive sport doing what will eventually mean anything of true worth within education and out in society at large?" Does it have anything like a "tenable theory" behind it to justify its presence in society at either the university or professional level? Sadly I must ask, "To what extent will it ever be possible to salvage what has become an increasingly out-of-control sport establishment?"

Middle schools, high schools, and colleges and universities need fine intramural and extramural sports and fitness programs. Do they have them? A small, indeterminate number of institutions do, but the large majority do not! We should be doing more to encourage the establishment of such programs and also to prepare fine sport and physical activity managers to administer them. I say: "Abolish overemphasized, commercialized sport—including the Olympic movement and now the new (ha!) 'extreme' sport fad."

Elementary and secondary educational institutions really need fine physical (activity) and health educators, not interscholastic sport coaches worrying about win-loss records that might threaten their tenure. We are finding increasingly that–somehow–many of these coaches have never been prepared *professionally* for the task. In addition, we cannot guarantee that they have been imbued with sound ethical perspectives in their "professional" environment.

Despite my extensive background in athletics and coaching, I have finally come to believe that the coaching of interscholastic athletics and inter–institutional athletics in higher education should be completely *separate* from the physical education unit in the respective institution. Today we are beginning to truly understand the crisis in regard to the fitness and health status of the large majority of youth. The welfare of these boys and girls *must* be paramount. Competitive sport for the "accelerated" should be promoted *only after* the welfare of all of our youths has been looked after adequately.

## Commercialized Sport Is Threatening Sport's Potential Value to Humankind!

Humankind's struggle to "make a go of it" in the twentieth century starkly outlined what now confronts humanity in the 21st century. Living together peacefully, of course, is an ever-present challenge of the highest magnitude. The great historian, Toynbee, reminded us that civilizations died when they simply did not confront challenges successfully. Climate change, for example, is rapidly developing into such a challenge, as are the ongoing clashes of unwavering religions.

There is another challenge, however. The world's populace does not seem to recognize that human involvement with sport is being characterized increasingly by overemphasis, commercialism, and violence as it "progresses professionally, technologically, and commercially." This now appears to have reached the point that it may be having a negative influence on society overall, as well as on the quality and quantity of the physical activity education programs of children and youth.

## Sporting Patterns Forged by Environmental Forces

Keep in mind the thought of Phyllis Hill cited above, in her insightful study (1965), titled *A Cultural History of Sport in Illinois*, 1673-1820. Recall that she concluded that the idea of "sport for sport's sake" is "inoperable" in a culture where sport is closely tied to personal achievement and success, and where work ethics and sport ethics are so close as to be virtually indistinguishable.

Hill explained further that, even though we complain about professionalism and the related conduct of athletes, we must remember that "halcyon amateurism" was never regarded as a value. In addition, American institutions became less and less tied to British tradition as the settlers moved west. Thus, she stressed that:

> The solution to American sporting problems does not lie in English tradition. Rather, sport in America is a cultural phenomenon, and its problems must be studied and resolved in the American tradition (1975).

Whatever the situation may be, sport has emerged as a universal social institution that was presumably designed originally to serve humankind by helping people to cope with an ever more complex societal life characterized by conflict and turmoil. As Hill stated, "Its problems must be studied and resolved in the American tradition." The question remains: How well is society or world culture accomplishing this purpose today?

As I discuss the situation today, having assumed increasingly a Cassandra-like mien that warns of increasing societal problems because of the way this proclivity to extreme commercialization and "technologizing" of sporting activity is heading, along with its increasing violence and added elements of danger, I can only conclude that it has become one of the world's major "blind spots". *This activity—presumably designed to serve humankind beneficially—may be doing just the opposite! In a variety of ways, the more complex and commercial it becomes, it is actually introducing beliefs and practices that influence participants and spectators negatively.*

Considering this matter more seriously, it appears that the "sport mentality of the United States is contributing significantly in the development of what may be regarded as the *socio-instrumental or material* values--that is, *the values of teamwork, loyalty, self-sacrifice, and perseverance consonant with prevailing corporate capitalism in democracy and in other political systems as well.* Conversely, however, we may also discover that there is now a great deal of evidence that sport may be developing *an ideal that also opposes the fundamental moral virtues of honesty, fairness, and responsibility in the innumerable competitive experiences provided* (Lumpkin, Stoll, and Beller, 1999).

Significant to this discussion are the results of investigations carried out by Hahm, Stoll, Beller, and Rudd. The Hahm-Beller Choice Inventory (HBVCI) has now been administered to athletes at different levels in a variety of venues. It demonstrates conclusively that athletes will not support what is considered "the moral ideal" in competition. As Stoll and Beller (1998) saw it, for example, an athlete with moral character demonstrates the moral character traits of honesty, fair play, respect, and responsibility whether an official is present to enforce the rules or not. Priest, Krause, and Beach (1999) reported, also, that--over a four-year period in a college athlete's career--ethical value choices showed decreases in "sportsmanship orientation" and an increase in "professional" attitudes associated with sport.

On the other hand, even though dictionaries define social character similarly, sport practitioners, including participants, coaches, parents, and officials, have come to believe that character is defined *properly* by such values as self-sacrifice, teamwork, loyalty, and perseverance mentioned above. The common expression in competitive sport is: "He/she showed character"--meaning "He/she 'hung in there' to the bitter end!" [or whatever]. Rudd (1999) confirmed that coaches explained character as "work ethic and commitment."

This coincides with what sport sociologists have found. Sage (1998. p. 614) stated that "Mottoes and slogans such as 'sports builds character' must be seen in the light of their ideological issues" In other words, competitive sport is structured by the nature of the society in which it occurs. This would appear to mean that over-commercialization, drug-taking, cheating, bribe-taking by officials, violence, etc. at all levels of sport are simply reflections of the culture in which we live. Where does that leave us today as we consider sport's presumed relationship with moral character development?

This discussion about whether sport's presumed educational and recreational roles have justification in fact could go on indefinitely. So many negative incidents have occurred that one hardly knows where to turn to avoid further negative examples. On the one hand we read the almost unbelievably high standards stated in the Code of Conduct developed by the Coaches Council of the National Association for Sport and Physical Education (2001). Conversely we learn that today athletes' concern for the presence of moral values in sport *declines* over the course of a university career (Priest, Krause, and Beach, 1999).

With this as a backdrop, we learn further that Americans, for example, are increasingly facing the cost and consequences of sedentary living (Booth & Chakravarthy, 2002). Additionally, Malina (2001) tells us that there is a need to track people's involvement in physical activity and sport across their life spans. Finally, Corbin and Pangrazi (2001) explain that we haven't yet been able to devise and accept a uniform definition of wellness for all people. The one thought that emerges from these various assessments is as follows: We give every evidence that we desire "sport spectaculars" for the few much more than we want people of all ages and all conditions to themselves have meaningful exercise involvement and recreational sport throughout their lives.

## Conceptualizing the Ritual of Sport

I then sought to conceptualize this time more precisely–that is, what the ritual of competitive sport should mean. I recalled that I had discussed the topic many years ago with the late Harry M. Johnson, Ph.D., of the University of Illinois, UIUC.

Johnson stressed that sport involvement was fundamentally meant to be connected with the all-important values of human life that, in slightly different forms, are vital for all "valuable' human activities. Among these values we concluded are the following:

1. Health itself (of course),

2. The value of trying to make a contribution regardless of actual success--the value of effort itself,

3. The value of actual achievement, including excellence,

4. The value of respect for opponents,

5. The value of cooperation (i.e., one's ability to subordinate the self to the attainment of collective goals),

6. The value of fair play (i.e., respect for the rules of competition, which are universal ideally),

7. The value of orderly procedure for the settling of disputes, and

8. The value of grace in intensively competitive situations--including magnanimity in victory and the ability to accept defeat gracefully--and then try to gain victory the next time.

To continue, there can be no doubt that the celebration of such values as these listed (immediately above) in competitive sport have this ritualistic quality described. We can arguably say this, because the immediate objectives and long-range goals of games, and what may be called educational and/or recreational sport, are presumably not intrinsically important. However, we have found that intrinsic importance may be given to them adventitiously causing them to become significant economic factors in society. The result of such "donation" has steadily and increasingly become an aberration threatening to become a negative social force impacting on societal wellbeing.

Basically, sport is said to be "pure" when the values are practiced and celebrated for their own sake as (for example) human love and a sense of community are celebrated in quite pure form in various civic ceremonies. Thus, when sport is "pure" in this sense, it presumably renews within the performers and knowledgeable spectators specific commitments to the very values that are being displayed and appreciated in public under relatively strict rules and surveillance. This type of display guarantees the noninterference of extraneous, unevenly distributed advantages.

In other words, the "purity" of ritual in both sport and many civic ceremonies should mean that certain social values are highlighted by being removed and protected from the distracting circumstances of everyday life--

handicaps and temptations as well as the inevitable involvement of immediately specific goals.

## The Ritual Inherent in Sport Competition
## *Must Not* Be Corrupted

Thus, careful analysis of the developing situation should be telling us that we must be most diligent in doing all that we can to see to it that the important ritual inherent in sport competition is not endangered, distorted, and corrupted–as it often is now under the following circumstances:
4

1. When so much emphasis is placed on winning, achievement of all the other values tends to be lost or negated.
2. When the financial rewards of advanced–level participation make sport predominantly a practical activity (rather than a ritual celebrating values for their own sake).
3. When competitive sport becomes largely entertainment for which the public pays "top dollar" so that team owners and competitors may be adequately compensated.

   (Note: Such competition increasingly involves the enjoyment of out-and-out brutality and even foul play rather than being a deeply serious and lastingly satisfying kind of activity [such as religious ritual itself is under the finest type of situation].)

4. When too sharp a separation is made between the performers and the spectators (consumers).

   (Note: In other words, the game (or religious ritual!) played or enacted before spectators as consumers needs to have a relationship to the "real life" activities of those who look on and/or partake.

5. When there is a loss of perspective, and skill of a physical nature and outstanding performance are made exclusive or the highest of values, we forget that these are largely instrumental

122

in nature.

*Thus, in addition to the valuable sport experience itself at the time, it is what these concurrent values are presumably required for subsequently that is truly important--that is, achievement off the playing field and enjoyment of a fine life experience through the medium of the sport contest and all that this could involve.*

Viewed in this way, a disinterested observer can say: "Yes, I do understand what relationship the right kind of involvement in sport and tangentially related physical activity has to the fundamental purpose of a society."

## The Ritual of Sport *Is* Being Corrupted

However, just what are we permitting to happen at present? The ritual of sport is being corrupted daily. The following is a list of our "transgressions" that could be easily expanded:

1. Promoting the idea that "**WINNING**" is the only thing…
2. Spending infinitely more money on varsity sports for the very few than that spent on intramural sports for the overwhelming majority
3. Offering "athletic scholarships" when there is no "financial need".
4. Permitting "trash talk" in competitive sport.
5. Permitting "showboating" by athletes after a successful play.
6. Permitting "TV sport universities" to debase education by promoting semi-professional sport played by so-called "scholar-athletes".
7. Permitting professional boxing (with the attendant brain damage!)
8. Featuring professional wrestling on television that is a disgusting sham and travesty of the fine sport of wrestling
9. Permitting "all-out" combat ("Extreme Sport") on television (and now it's offered for women too!).
10. Permitting (promoting?) the development of "high-risk" sport where "life and limb" are increasingly threatened.
11. Promoting the idea that competitive sport is good for young people, but then denying funding for intramural sport for the large majority of students in the schools.

12. Permitting professional boxing as a sport for women too!
13. Encouraging the whole idea of "martial-art" sport–when it's "self-defense" that should be stressed—not aggression!
14. Failing to take action sooner--and more strongly!– against drugs in sport. This abuse will "kill" sport in the long run… (Is this the antidote?)
15. Permitting the type of sport in which studies have shown *fair play, honesty, and sportsmanship actually decline in a university experience* (Stoll et al.).
16. Paying ridiculously high salaries to professional athletes thus creating a "false sense of values" to youth.
17. Permitting the concept of "hero" to be applied to professional athletes unworthy of such ascription, thus unduly influencing youth as to what's important in life.
18. Overemphasizing the importance of involvement (*and winning!*) in *international* sport competition. (the "Own the podium" mentality)
19. Permitting the expansion of "violent" sports, but not also making appropriate provisions for excellent "sport injury care" for all.
20. Fostering a way of life that encourages "spectatoritis" instead of actual ongoing involvement in healthful physical activity and sport.

## The Appropriate Remedies for "Errant" Sport Must Be Instituted

If these conditions are true, it means that we need to assess the evolving situation carefully and then proceed to institute the appropriate remedies. To provide us with an approach that should help to communicate with policy makers at all levels about this ever-increasing problem, consider the five–question approach to the building of effective communication skills recommended by Mark Bowden, a communications specialist (*National Post*, Canada, 2008 11 24, FP3)

*Question 1: Where are we now?*

The answer is that we have in so many instances permitted deviation from the basic, valuable purposes for which sport was originally created. Osterhoudt (2006) tells us that competitive sport has become increasingly devoted to "the production, distribution, and consumption of commodities, power, wealth, fame, and privilege in predominantly medical, military, character enhancement, acculturative, political, commercial, entertainment, and recreational terms, which is to say in *instrumental* terms" (R. G. Osterhoudt in *Sport As a Form of Human Fulfillment,* Victoria, BC, CA: Trafford, 2006)).

*Question 2. Why are we here?*

The answer is that we are here because society has mistakenly permitted the excess of capitalistic and technological development to influence and adversely affect sport in the same way that other societal institutions have been affected by these developments. Sport does indeed seem to be "the opiate of the masses"! Such development and "progress" have also joined forces with ongoing technological advancement confronting society almost irresistibly and irrevocably.

*Question 3. Where do we want to be?*

The answer is—as mentioned above—that we want to make certain that we create a situation where *"Sport involvement is related to and connected with the all-important values of human life that, in slightly different forms, are vital for all 'valuable' human activities."*

*Question 4. How do we get there?*

The answer is that we get there by seeing to it, therefore, that *the important ritual inherent in sport competition* is maintained to the greatest extent possible. As we have seen, it has been endangered, distorted, and corrupted by the presence of the following circumstances:

> a. When so much emphasis is placed on winning, achievement of all the other values tends to be lost or negated.
> b. When the financial rewards of advanced-level participation make sport predominantly a practical activity (rather than a ritual celebrating values for their

125

own sake).

c. When competitive sport becomes largely
   entertainment for which the public
   pays "top dollar" so that team owners and
   competitors may be adequately compensated.

(Note: Such competition increasingly involves the enjoyment of
out-and-out brutality and even foul play rather than being a
deeply serious and lastingly satisfying kind of activity.)

d. When too sharp a separation is made between
   the performers and the spectators (consumers).

(Note: In other words, the game or context that
is played or enacted before spectators [i.e.,
consumers] needs to have a relationship to the
"real life" activities of those who look on
and/or partake.

e. When there is a loss of perspective, and
   skill of a physical nature and outstanding performance
   are made exclusive or the highest of values, we forget
   that these are largely *instrumental* in nature for the
   achievement of power, wealth, fame, and privilege in
   predominantly commercial and entertainment
   enterprises.

*Thus, it is what these values are presumably required for*
*subsequently is what's really important--that is, achievement*
*off the playing field and enjoyment of a fine life experience*
*through the medium of the sport contest and all that this could involve.*

*Question 5. What exactly should we do?*

The answer is that we should encourage all professionals
active in physical activity education and educational sport to
place *quality* as the first priority of their professional endeavors. Their
personal involvement and specialization should include a high level of
competency and skill under girded by established knowledge about the
highest type of aims and objectives in competitive sport that our field should
be promoting. On such a basis, it can be argued that the role of physical

activity educators (including sport coaches is as important as any in society.

## Is Competitive Sport Doing More Good Than Harm?

The professional sport management associations, established relatively recently nationally and internationally, have a unique opportunity to exert at least some influence on the future of sport through their efforts in sport management education in society generally. Looking to this end, I offer several thoughts for you to consider. I believe we need to truly understand "where sport has been" and "where it is now" if we ever hope to know "where sport should go."

I believe we should be able to prove that sport as a social institution is doing more good than harm in society. Right now I have the uneasy feeling that this may not be so. It is up to those socio-cultural scholars and scientists in our midst to develop an increasing amount of sound theory backed by field-tested investigation. Additionally, there is a need for solid theory about sport and physical activity *management* itself. The blossoming sport management profession should prove to the world that sport is doing what its adherents purports that it does. We actually need an ongoing scientific inventory of ordered generalizations about (a) what we know and (b) what we think we know about the physical activity experience in competitive sport (being careful to separate the "a" and "b" categories).

## Concluding Statement

Finally, there are those who say that America is in decline, and that overemphasized sport itself contributes to the accuracy of this assertion. I can only say to those interested in sport management professionally, semi-professionally, or even on a voluntary basis: "Ladies and gentlemen--even though the 'multitude out there'--and, indeed, many of us—may not appreciate it, sport as a social institution does appear to have gradually but steadily been influenced negatively by the declining value structure of society." Hence, it is up to us to make a case more strongly so that society will guarantee that children and youth have the *finest* type of sport experience. Sport itself has developed to such an extent that it has become a social force–an institution!–that could have a beneficial effect on society overall if we only permit and encourage it to do so.

The present is no time for indecision, half-hearted commitment, imprecise knowledge, and general unwillingness to debate this position about the highest or ideal form of sport participation with the public at all levels. If we hope to bring the

127

benefits of the "*right* kind" of sport participation to children and youth, we must sharpen our focus and improve the quality of our professional effort. Only in this way will we be able to combat the modification process that capitalistic society and accompanying technology have visited upon us in respect to people's understanding of what constitutes the finest type of competitive sport. In the 21st century, humankind deserves better than the type of sport as a social institution that "somehow!" gradually materialized in the 20th century.

# Chapter 8
# Examples of the Kaleidoscopic Value Orientation
# (1) of Sport in the Public Sector
# & (2) of Physical Activity Education Within Education

In Part 8 I have included a number of examples depicting the developing kaleidoscopic value orientation of the problems and concerns related to human physical activity in exercise, sport, dance, and physical recreation at all levels and in the public sector. My position is that, individually and collectively, instances such as these serve to "make the case" that the present situation is becoming steadily and increasingly undesirable as we look to the future in the 21st century.

In describing competitive sport in the public sector, it could be classified as amateur, semiprofessional or professional, but somehow the distinction has become ever more "blurred". The category "semiprofessional" is present in practice, but it has never been "officially recognized". Compared to the standards set in their ethical codes for practitioners by the established professions (e.g., education, law, medicine) the only thing that seems to be truly professional about sport in most circumstances is the fact that the participants receive money for their services! In addition, a number of them receive ridiculously high amounts of that legal tender.

In the case of physical (activity) education, however, teachers become members of the education profession, have university degrees, and must be licensed to teach in public education. The problem here is that, despite the mounting of irrefutable evidence as to the benefits of regular exercise and physical recreation through intramural athletics, instruction for "normal" and "special-needs" children and youth, the program mandated in states and provinces varies consistently from good, to fair, to poor, to "non-existent"! The "varsity sport program" for the very few, however, is typically "good" to "excellent."

## Sport as an Anti-value?

To continue, the basic argument being presented here is as fellows: *unless sport participation does "such-and-such" to make people and the society in which they live a better place, such instances must simply be regarded as serving as anti-values!*

What we are finding increasingly is a situation where people seem to be so anxious to escape the *real* world that they are rushing into various sports and similar activities with increasing intensity seemingly unaware of the dangers and the potential outcomes of such involvement. (One wonders where the parents are in such instances…)

Coincidently, onrushing science and technology have also become *the tempters of many coaches and athletes*. This possibility has added another dimension to the personal and professional conduct of those people who are unduly anxious for recognition and financial gain.

The premise presented here is, therefore, that beliefs such as these have created a vacuum of positive belief. Hence, sport is overall increasingly becoming more of an anti-value for those who would view **educational co**mpetitive sport as a *life-enhancer* (e.g., those interuniversity sports that are not sustained through gate receipts--golf, tennis, wrestling, swimming, gymnastics, soccer, and almost all of women's sport).

Thus, in an effort to build on Chapter 7 that discussed "what went wrong in the 20th century", Chapter 8 includes a kaleidoscope of items that supplement and enhance the claims made in Part 7.

## Physical Education As "All Things to All People" or "Not Too Much To Anyone"

Shifting attention to the exercise component and the intramural athletics component of the overall physical activity program (including varsity competitive sport), the development of what was originally the Association for the Advance of Physical Education (with the word "American" added the next year) has been interesting and successful in a variety of ways depending on the interpretation of the word "success." Physical education has been termed a profession, but it really is a field within the profession of education. Unfortunately, somehow the connotation of the name–and it reduction to "PE"–is such that it was not (could not be) used as the name for a profession outside of the educational establishment in the public sector.

Subsequently within the Association, however, a number of so-called "allied" professions" emerged (i.e., health education, safety education, recreation and park administration, dance (education), athletics (sport), and exercise therapy). The development of these "professions" was undoubtedly influenced down through the years by social forces or societal influences of greater or lesser intensity.

Hess (1959) helped us to somewhat understand how what happened socially and politically enabled him to delineate the leading objectives of physical education from 1900 to 1960:

Hygiene or Health Objective–1900-1919
Socio-Educational Objective–1920-1929
Socio-Recreational Objective–1930-1939
Physical Fitness & Health Objective–1939-1945
'Total Fitness' and International Understanding–
    1946-1957
Disciplinary Development–1959-???

While all of this socio-political development was occurring, a succession of leaders in the field of physical education were attempting to spell out their visions of the field's objectives in the literature. The following is a chronological list of these leading scholars/practitioners from 1900 to 1950 (see References and Bibliography below, also).:

Hetherington, Wood and Cassidy, Williams, Hughes, Bowen and Mitchell, Nash, Sharman, Wayman.
Esslinger, Staley, McCloy, Clark, Cobb, Lynn, Brownell
Scott, Bucher, Oberteuffer, Metheny, Shepherd, Brightbill, Sapora.

An analysis of their recommendations (Zeigler, 1977) resulted on a listing of what might be called "common denominators" in program development:

Movement Fundamentals
Regular Exercise
Health & Safety Education
Physical Recreation
Physical Fitness
Competitive Sport
Therapeutic Exercise

Now I have expanded a bit on this list of so-called "common denominators" for physical activity education in the hope that there might be considerable agreement in the developed world. These proposed common denominators are as follows:

1. That regular physical activity education (including related health information) be *required* for all children and young people up to and including sixteen years of age.
2. That human movement fundamentals through various dance and other expressive activities be included in the elementary, middle, and high school curricula.
3. That progressive standards for physical vigor and endurance for people of all ages be developed from prevailing norms.
4. That the physical activity & health educator's responsibility should be *a full-time one*.

> (**Note:** The implication here is that any sport coaching involvement on his or her part would be the same as that with any other teacher in the school based on the practices of the community involved.)

5. That remediable bodily defects be corrected where possible through exercise therapy. Referral to the family doctor may be necessary to initiate a remedial program. Where possible, adapted sport and physical recreation experiences should be offered.
6. That boys and girls (and young men and women) have an experience in competitive sport at some stage of their development.
7. That people develop certain positive attitudes toward their own health in particular and toward community hygiene in general. Basic health knowledge should be integral part of the school curriculum.

> (**Note:** This "common denominator" should be a specific objective of the profession of physical activity education only to the extent that it relates to developmental physical activity.)

8. That sport, dance, exercise, and play can make a most important contribution throughout life toward the worthy use of leisure.
9. That character and/or personality development is vitally important to the development of the young person. Therefore, it is especially important that all human movement experience in sport, dance, exercise, and play at the various educational levels be guided by men and women with high professional standards and ethics.

Despite the above, there is ongoing evidence that "all is not well." In 2006 Eleanor Randolph, in "The Big, Fat American Kid Crisis…and Things We Should Do About It" explained that:

The problem is all too obvious. At the mall, the movie theater or the airport, the evidence appears in the flesh – altogether too much of it. Americans are now officially supersized, overweight, obese even. This is true of almost two thirds of American adults, but what is more alarming, it is also true of millions of American children. The "little ones" aren't so little any more.

Yes, they are gent! labeled "chunky," "husky" or "plus-sized" by the clothes marketers who are adding larger and larger sizes to the children's racks. But these euphemisms can't cover up the unpleasant reality that too many of our kids are so dangerously overweight that they are spilling out of their childhood too chubby for their car seats or too uncomfortable as they squeeze into their little desks at elementary school. But the real problem is not aesthetics or the need to save classroom space. Childhood obesity has become a national medical crisis.

Over the last 30 years, obesity rates have doubled among pre-schoolers and tripled for those age 6 to 11. For those added pounds, the young are starting to pay a terrible price. Adult diabetes has rapidly become a childhood disease. Pediatricians are seeing high cholesterol and high blood pressure and other grown-up problems in their patients. Teachers and school psychiatrists are coping with a plague of shame and distress among children whose size subjects them to hazing and other cruelties by their classmates.

There is some evidence that more people are becoming aware of the two problems I have been describing. *The Wall Street Journal* (2010 06 09) summarized a report emanating from the National Association for Sport and Physical Education and the American Heart Association stating that there was a slight improvement in the percentage of states requiring physical education since that of a survey carried out in 2006. *However, most of the states have no requirement as to the time allotment of such a requirement—and half of them permits waivers, exemptions, and substitutions…"*

Reports of this type could go on endlessly, but I'll end with a conclusion stated in *Active Living Research*, a national program of the Robert Wood Johnson Foundation (Fall, 2007, Research Brief):

In schools across the United States, physical education has been substantially reduced—and in some cases completely eliminated—in response to budget concerns and pressures to improve academic test scores. Yet the available evidence shows that children who are physically active and fit tend to perform better in the classroom, and that daily physical education does not adversely affect academic performance. Schools can provide outstanding learning environments while improving children's health through physical education.

The situation in Canada doesn't appear to be much better. Jo-Ann Fellows, a columnist in Fredericton, NB, Canada, writes:

> For the fourth year in a row, a failing grade has been handed out to the whole country. Only 12 per cent of Canadian children and youth are meeting the guideline of 90 minutes per day.
>
> The report card was issued by Active Healthy Kids Canada. Its mandate states that it provides "... the evidence base for our communications and issue advocacy work to increase support for quality, accessible and enjoyable physical activity participation experiences for young people across Canada.

Following these brief analyses of the prevailing situation in public-sector sport and physical (activity) education (including sport) within the education establishment, I have included a number of examples to support the overall position being taken here.

## Example #1 (Professional Sport): Mixed Martial Arts Is a Mixed Bag

What has appeared in certain venues and on television is hardly what should be glorified in a civilized society. The goal in any so-called "sport" should not be to destroy your opponent literally.

However, the veneer of civilization is thin. At any given moment you may be called upon to defend yourself or some loved one. This tells you that *you should be prepared to defend yourself or a loved one at any given moment.* This dictum applies to both boys and girls *and to* men and women!

Yet, where do you acquire this knowledge and skill in today's society? The logical place for such acquisition would seem to be early on in a quality physical activity education program within the educational system. Good luck! Everything seems to have priority over this important educational program, much less training in self defense.

Above I stated: "mixed martial arts is a mixed bag." I stand by this statement. Learning self defense should be a vital, compulsory experience for all young people. Such competency could be acquired through amateur wrestling instruction within a physical activity education program for both boys and girls. Along the way, it is easy to explain how certain "dirty," illegal tactics could be used to disable an opponent.

"What about boxing instruction?" you may ask? This "sport" has been around for a long time, and could be helpful in self defense. However, it has been eliminated in educational institutions. I don't recommend it. As you train for this activity, the head is the primary target. Any brain surgeon will tell you how bad this is… For this reason alone, even though protective headgear helps, boxing should be banned at all levels.

Further, there are a variety of so-called martial–arts programs out there that have been imported from various world societies (e.g., karate and kung fu). The primary source for them is through private, commercial enterprises that require greater or lesser monetary expenditures. It is difficult to know which are the good or acceptable establishments. This means that a parent should discuss this matter with friends and neighbors, and also actually observe a variety of such offerings very carefully before signing any agreement to take part over a period of time.

This is why I recommend amateur wrestling instruction in physical activity education classes or as intramural and extramural sport. (I stress the word "amateur" because "professional" wrestling is nothing but vulgar, disgusting theater.) As a boy or girl acquires competency in amateur wrestling, it is easy to see how you can do "illegal things" and really hurt a person. The transition from "legal to illegal" is ever present.

If you are faced with a situation where you must defend yourself, you should know *automatically* how to carry out the illegal move or tactic to defend yourself if required. This knowledge and skill must be learned through practice and actual competition. Yet we can't risk hurting or maiming the participant in the process. It is a "tricky balance" that should be attained and maintained.

Good physical activity education includes instruction in body mechanics, physical fitness, leisure skills, aquatic ability, and self-defense. The first three competencies help one to lead a good life. Aquatic ability and competency in self defense can save your life.

Pick your mixed martial art most carefully. I recommend "supplemented" amateur wrestling for self defense.

## Example #2 (The Olympic Movement): On What Basis Should a Country Sponsor the Olympic Games?

There's a vocal minority who believe the Olympic Games should be abolished. There's another minority, including the Games officials and the athletes, who presumably feel the enterprise is doing just fine. There's a larger minority undoubtedly solidly behind the commercial aspects of the undertaking. They have a good thing going; they liked the Games the way they are developing--the bigger, the better! Finally, there's the vast majority to whom the Olympics are either interesting, somewhat interesting, or a bore. This "vast majority," if the Games weren't there every four years, would probably agree that the world would go on just the same, and some other social phenomenon would take up their leisure time.

The people love a spectacle. The 2000 Olympic Games held in Sydney, Australia were a spectacle, from start to finish. Sydney, Australia evidently wanted worldwide recognition. Without doubt, Sydney got recognition! The world's outstanding athletes wanted the opportunity to demonstrate their excellence. From all reports they had such an occasion to their heart's and ability's content. The International Olympic Committee, along with their counterparts in each of the 200 participating nations, earnestly desired the show to go on; it went on with a bang! Obviously, Sydney spent an enormous amount of money and energy to finance and otherwise support this extravaganza and surrounding competition. The IOC and its affiliates will presumably remain solvent for another four years, while Sydney contemplates its involvement with this enormous event and its aftermath.

"Problem, what problem?" most people in the public sector would assuredly ask if they were confronted with such a question..

*The Problem*

This analysis revolves around the criticisms of the "abolish the Games group." Sir William Rees-Mogg (1988, pp. 7-8), is one of the Olympic Movement's most vituperative opponents. He believes the problem is of enormous magnitude. In fact, he lists fifteen subproblems in no particular order of importance except for the first criticism that sets the tone for the remainder: "The Olympic Games have become a grotesque jamboree of international hypocrisy. Whatever idealism they once had has been lost. The Games now stand for some of the things which are most rotten and corrupt in the modern world, for prestige, nationalism, publicity, prejudice, bureaucracy, and the exploitation of talent" (p. 7).

It would not be appropriate to enumerate here *in great detail* the remaining 14 problems and issues brought forward by Rees-Mogg. Simply put, however, he states that "The Games have been taken over by a vulgar nationalism, in place of the spirit of internationalism for which they were revived" (p.7). He decries also that, in addition to promoting racial intolerance, "the objectives of many national Olympic programmes is the glorification and self-assertion of totalitarian state regimes," often "vile regimes guilty of many of the crimes which the Olympic Games are supposed to outlaw" (p. 7).

Rees-Mogg decries further "The administration of the Olympic Games [that] is politically influenced and morally bankrupt" (p. 7). Additionally, at this point, he asserts that "the international bureaucracies of several sports have become among the most odious of the world." In this respect he lashes out especially at tennis, chess, cricket, and track and field. Still further, he charges that threats by countries to boycott the Olympics have time and again made it a political arena akin to the United Nations.

The messenger has not yet completed his message. Rees-Mogg condemns "the worship of professionally abnormal muscular development," and states that it is "a form of idolatry to which ordinary life is often sacrificed" (p. 7). Since these words were written in 1988, these problems have assuredly not been corrected. They have actually worsened (e.g., ever-more drugs to enhance performance, bribery of officials assigned to site selection). The entire problem of drug ingestion to promote bodily development for enhanced performance has now become legendary. Couple this with over-training begun at early ages in selected sports for both boys and girls, and it can be argued safely that *natural* , all-round development has been thwarted for a great many young people, not to mention the fact that only a minute number makes it through to "Olympic glory." More could be said, but the point has been made. Basically, Rees-Mogg has claimed that it has become a world "in which good *values* are taken by dishonest men and put to shameful uses" (p. 8).

*An Assessment of the Problem.*

The problem, the author believes, is this: opportunities for participation in all competitive sport--not just *Olympic* sport-- moved historically from amateurism to semi-professionalism, and then on to full-blown professionalism. The Olympic Movement, because of a variety of social pressures, followed suit in both ancient times and in the present. When the International Olympic Committee gave that final push to the pendulum and openly admitted professional athletes to play in the Games, they may have pleased most of the spectators and all of the advertising and media representatives. But in so doing the floodgates were opened completely, and the original ideals upon which the Games were reactivated were completely abandoned. This is what caused Sir Rees-Mogg to state that crass commercialism had won the day. This final abandonment of any semblance of what was the original Olympic ideal was the "straw that broke the camel's back." This ultimate decision regarding eligibility for participation has indeed been devastating to those people who earnestly believe that money and sport are like oil and water; they simply do not mix! Their response has been to abandon any further interest in, or support for, the entire Olympic Movement.

The question must, therefore be asked: "What should rampant professionalism in competitive sport at the Olympic Games mean to any given country out of the 200 nations involved?" This is not a simple question to answer responsibly. In this present brief statement, it should be made clear that the professed social values of a country *should* ultimately prevail--and they *will* prevail in the final analysis. However, this ultimate determination will not take place overnight. The *fundamental social values* of a social system will eventually have a strong influence on the *individual values* held by most citizens in that country, also. If a country is moving toward the most important twin values of equalitarianism and achievement, for example, what implications does that have for competitive sport in that political entity under consideration? The following are some questions that should be asked *before* a strong continuing commitment is made to sponsor such involvement through governmental and/or private funding:

138

1. *Can it be shown that* involvement in competitive sport atone or the other of the three levels (i.e., amateur, semiprofessional, professional) brings about desirable *social* values (i.e., more valuethan disvalue)?

2. *Can it be shown that* involvement in competitive sport at one or the other of the three levels (i.e., amateur, semiprofessional, or professional) brings about desirable *individual* values of both an *intrinsic* and *extrinsic* nature (i.e., creates more value than disvalue)?

3. *If the answer to Questions #1 amd #2 immediately are both affirmative* (i.e., that involvement in competitive sport at any or all of the three levels postulated [i.e., *amateur, semiprofessional, and professional* sport] provides a sufficient amount of social and individual value to warrant such promotion), can sufficient funds be made available to support or permit this promotion atany or all of the three levels listed?

4. *If funding to support participation in competitive sport at any or all of the three levels (amateur, semiprofessional, professional) is not available (or such participation is not deemed advisable), should priorities--as determined by the expressed will of the people--be established about the importance of each level to the country based on careful analysis of the potential social and individual values that may accrue to the society and its citizens from such competitive sport participation at one or more levels?*

*Concluding Statement*

    In this analysis the investigator asks whether a country should be involved with, or continue involvement with, the ongoing Olympic Movement--as well as *all* competitive sport--unless the people in that country first answer some basic questions. These questions ask to what extent such involvement can be related to the social and individual values that the country holds as important for all of its citizens. Initially, study will be needed to determine whether sport competition at either or all of the three levels (i.e., amateur, semi-professional, and professional) does indeed provide positive social and individual value (i.e., more value than disvalue) in the country concerned. Then careful assessment--through the efforts of qualified social scientists and philosophers--should be made of the populace's opinions and basic beliefs about such involvement. If participation in competitive sport at each of the three levels can make this claim to being a social institution that provides positive value to the country, these efforts should be supported to the extent possible--including the sending of a team to future Olympic Games. If sufficient funding for the support of *all* three levels of participation is *not* available, from either governmental or private sources, *the expressed will of the people should be established to determine what priorities will be invoked.*

**Example #3 (Intercollegiate Athletics):**
**What Price Glory in Intercollegiate Football:**
**(Siwash "U" in the Mid–50s)**

> Note: The names and places in this example have been altered to preserve anonymity.

This brief story is a factual case about the football fortunes of a well-known football power in the United States 50 years ago. All proper names have been changed to avoid embarrassment to anyone involved in the program at that time (i.e., to protect both the innocent and the guilty). The basic material was taken almost completely from several national magazines, local newspapers, personal letters from close observers, and observations of associates. The sources cannot be revealed.)

There was a time when the blue-and-gold uniforms of the Bears were an ominous sight in the Northern State Conference. During the days of old Sam Jackson (1908-16), when many colleges were still playing rugby, the State University of Siwash never lost a football game. After World War I, Jack Thompson, a rugged homegrown coach, built a formidable series of teams out of the big youths in their native region. Players like Lars Larson and the fabled Jordan brothers led Siwash into the Camelia Bowl after the 1923 and 1935 seasons, the golden era of Siwash University football. Like Larson, SU backs seemed to run over rather than around anyone brave enough to get in their way. They were truly the Bears of football.

It was symbolic of Siwash football that "hometowners" considered it sissy stuff when the college put turf on the home stadium after the arrival of Coach Jim Jenkins in 1930. The hides of the home players were so tough they had never been bothered by the sand-and-gravel surface that sent visiting teams away whining in pain. With the advent of grass there was a long dry spell in Bear football, punctured by only one Camelia Bowl visit--in 1937, when Rand State U. walloped them 21-0. Not until Burt Sanderson and Jon Blake, later to star as pros, brightened up the team in the early 1950s did Bear rooters have anything to root about, but their cheers were brief. The simple fact was that all the best SU football talent was coming from adjoining states, where Sanderson had been discovered, and Siwash wasn't getting its fair share any more.

Joe Briggs stepped into this football void in 1953 with a huge local reputation. From 1930-32 he had been a Bear backfield star, winner in his senior year of the Standlee Medal as the "most inspirational player." Later as a high school coach in Suffridge, he had stepped out and won three championships. Then, as the Bear freshman coach for five years, his teams won 22 out of 23. So, when Coach George Graham went down the chute after a 7-3 win-loss season, the cry for Briggs was too loud to be denied. Bob Golden, the Gridiron Club president, Athletic Director Hanley Borden, and at least one member of the University board of trustees, would have preferred former Backfield Coach Rock Steckel (now at Jordan U.), but the alumni would not be denied. Briggs was hired.

Good football players, to put it mildly, are not easy to come by. A good team can cost $5,000 a month or more in scholarships and campus-job payments, and, when that isn't sufficient, special inducements such as convertibles and free trips home and vacation jobs and even jobs for the players' wives. Football players, if they are smart enough to learn a fake reverse, understand their own value and are quick to capitalize on it.

No one knows this better than Bob Golden, president of the Gridiron Club and a really remarkable booster in a city of boosters. Since his undergraduate days at Siwash, Bob Golden, a carrot-topped little dynamo who was a .300-hitting second baseman on the college team and president of the Big S club in his senior year, has been all for the Bears. Right after graduation in 1923, as assistant graduate manager, he started working for better football, and he doesn't mind admitting that he helped build the Camelia Bowl teams of 1924 and 1926. Nowadays Bob is Mr. Football around Siwash, and it was he that much of the conversation concerned last week.

So that good football players may enjoy the advantages of a Siwash U education, Bob Golden runs the Siwash Advertising Fund, which, as he tells it, is used "primarily for transportation costs, entertainment, and expenses for prospective athletes." Once Bob explained: "It's a fact of life that a kid can't be a college athlete and make it through school if he's in any need at all without outside help, and that's why there's a fund like ours at almost every other university."

Bob's fund is a big one--it has run in the past anywhere from $20,000 to $75,000--and he runs it pretty much as he pleases. Mostly the contributions come from 70 to 80 local big and little businessmen, labor leaders, medical doctors, lawyers, and others interested in civic betterment, people who contributed checks ranging up from fifty dollars. Now and then Bob sees a chance to make an extra pile for the fund, such as the exhibition pro football game last summer held in Siwash Stadium. The Advertising Fund netted $28,000 for this effort.

Everyone, particularly university and state officials, seems very surprised with this piece of information when it was finally published. No one pretended there was anything dishonest about it. They just seemed surprised that what had passed for an event to greaten the city of Siwash--and a *professional* sports event at that--was helping put amateur football players through the local university. No doubt if they had been told about it in advance, they would have been perfectly happy. Hearing about it later was something of a shock.

Coach Joe Briggs, who was appointed in 1953, is a man who inspires fierce loyalty among his friends. Nonetheless, even by his own appraisal, he is not an easy man to be with. "I've been told I'm sarcastic, and I admit it," he said recently. "I bore down on the kids during the week so they'd be prepared for the pressure on Saturday. I goaded the kids and I needled them and I demanded discipline. I wanted Saturday to seem like a breeze to them. Let's not kid each other; there's not enough discipline anywhere today for modern kids. I think football is the last frontier of discipline."

Like any coach, Joe had his share--perhaps more--of bad luck in his first two years. There were injuries to key players at the worst time, and there were vital plays called back for penalties. Yet his real problem was that of most losing coaches, lack of good manpower. As a result he won only five of his first 20 games. Once, on a road trip to Stanton, Joe was visited at a practice session by Rex Louth, his old Bear coach, now retired. Louth watched for a while, then said: "Joe, you better get some ballplayers. You haven't got a guy on that field who's worth a newspaper photographer's time."

This was no news to Briggs, or to Golden or any of the other Bear boosters, of whom even faraway southern Dyckstra has its share. The most active of them in that area, a clique that revolves around Stanton, soon stole some of the cream of the Stanton area junior colleges right out from under the noses of such football powers as Stanton and Boulder. It was quite a haul, but as a Stanton booster observed about Siwash: "When they want a man, they get him. They dig."

142

Not the least of Siwash's athletic harvest was Reg Branch, who had coached the great Sid Tanzer at Waterloo High School. Originally Branch had left Waterloo to go to Stanton along with Sid in what the cognoscenti call a "package deal." However, when Sid became unhappy and defected to Boulder, Branch was nevertheless kept on for another year despite his frequent criticisms of Head Coach Sands' methods to other assistant coaches. So, when Siwash hired Branch as an assistant for Briggs last spring, Branch was given an enthusiastic farewell by his fellow coaches at Stanton. For Siwash he presumably represented an attraction and a pipeline to top high school players in the Stanton area.

Branch did indeed help Briggs and his assistants come up with a good crop of recruits including some excellent junior college transfers. So, when the Bear varsity lined up against ineffectual little Statler University last September 17 for an easy opener, it was obvious to anyone who knew the ABC's of football in Siwash that this was the make-or-break year for Joe Briggs. As the game progressed, however, Briggs could hardly believe his eyes. The team fumbled 11 times for a new conference record and barely eked out a 14-7 victory. Not until the coaches had studied the game film, however, did they discover that the center had been snapping the ball a half-count too soon. Some quick detective work revealed that he had done so on the instructions of one Reg Branch. "I was just trying an experiment," Branch explained. "I wanted to fire Branch on the spot," responded Briggs, "but Hanley Borden, our AD, advised me to wait."

For a while the Bears seemed to have regained their poise, rolling over Sparland 30-0 and upsetting powerful Boulder 7-0. Then followed two very mediocre weeks against Lanier and Douglas, and finally defeats by Lockland State and Stanton. By this time it was obvious something was terribly wrong. "I find out," stated Briggs, "that Marshall [quarterback Topper Marshall, a demoted first-stringer] is trying to persuad the most promising young quarterback on the squad to leave school. I bounced Marshall off the squad, but I wound up taking him back when [booster] Golden played sweet music on my heart strings by telling me that Marshall would lose his sponsor and also be evicted from his home. So, after he apologized to the squad, I took him back, but he went right on spreading dissension."

The first explosion came at the end of the season when a group of Bear players marched in to see Bob Golden to complain of Joe Briggs's coaching. They had signed a petition asking for his release. The coach, they said, was too strict; he would not let them ride home from games with their girlfriends; he yelled at them; he would not let them whistle in the dressing room or chew grass (!); and he made them sit erect on the bench. Citing a list of these and other complaints, the players stated that four promising freshmen had quite Siwash to solicit offers elsewhere.

Golden passed the list of complaints along to the athletic director, Hanley Borden, who passed the complaint along to the board of trustees. After a lengthy meeting, Briggs was rehired with the injunction to "straighten out his differences with his players." Anyone who knew Siwash football could have told you that Joe Briggs was through. He buried the hatchet and smoked a peace pipe with most of his players, but he was still out of grace with both Borden and Golden. What he could not patch up was his 5-4-1 record. (It is interesting to note that at the time of the revolt and the petition, pro-Briggs squad members suddenly found their mailbags empty of checks. "Players," said Joe, "had to look in two directions: one way for favors, the other for coaching."

Briggs received a late Xmas present--he was fired on January 27. The next day he started to talk to any and all who would listen. His righteous indignation was bursting out all over. "The filthiest thing in the world," he said, "is to corrupt young Americans with dough. I may never coach again, but, God willing, I'm not going to let them corrupt any more kids." Later he added: "I went along, all right-- with the full knowledge of my superiors. No coach has any other choice under the unrealistic rules that prevail in the Western State Conference and others like it."

Interestingly, everyone else around the campus seemed quite stunned at the thought that football players were receiving extracurricular salaries. Said AD Hanley Borden: "To the best of my knowledge, no coach or myself has at any time willfully violated the conference rules. Neither I nor any member of my department has had any relationship with any so-called fund."

The president of Siwash, the eminent Harlow Standish, echoed the denial: "I want to say at once that these suggestions simply are not true." A re-echo came from Vice-President R.A. (Rick) Allen, a former president of the Western State Conference, who announced: "Were I to receive evidence that any player has been receiving anything like outside monthly payments, I would immediately declare him disqualified for team participation." The Board of Trustees? Said its chair, Mrs. R. Douglas Smythe, who with her husband, a financial consultant, are long-time friends of Hanley Borden: "I know nothing about it at all."

144

## Example #4 (Clash of Moral and
### Socio-Instrumental Values):
## Tiger Woods Is Caught in a Vise:

*The Occurrence.* Tiger Woods, named the outstanding golf professional of the 2000-2009 decade and undoubtedly a "golden boy" in the sporting world, has been leading a double life. Presumably happily married to a beautiful Swedish wife with two lovely children, and on the way to becoming fabulously wealthy, Woods had an automobile accident outside of his home in the early hours of a morning. This mishap subsequently brought to light a tale of extraordinary, "extracurricular" sexual activity with many mistresses far and wide.

This scandal immediately became one of the top media stories of the year 2009. The public was surprised and also startled. In fairly short order, the "miscreant" felt constrained to offer a public apology and to take an indefinite leave from his work as professional gold player. The implications resulting from this move away from the "world of golf" were potentially devastating to both the future of Woods himself and to the development of the sport of golf.

*Why Was This Story So Newsworthy?* Watching this scandal mature over several months, I asked myself: "Why was this such a 'big deal'?" Is this development so unusual in the history of the world? Haven't various media personalities, including sport figures, experienced problems of this type before? Why is this particular incident worthy of all this attention? (*Note:* The ethical aspect of his relationship with Dr. Galea in Toronto who administered PEDs in Toronto to speed up Tiger's recovery from knee surgery is not considered here.) The answer is that this incident is not *unique*, but it is *unusual.* Yet, one wonders why has so much public attention been given to this particular situation? I believe the answer can be found in the fact that, over the past one hundred years, the role of sport in society has changed most radically. Competitive sport has gradually, but steadily, become a *social institution* that somehow because of capitalism, politics, and money surged enormously in importance. Hence, it has become an extremely powerful social force that must be reckoned with from here into the indeterminate future.

Because of this upsurge in sport's development, I have personally been attempting to analyze it from a socio-cultural perspective. It appears to be a question of the "use of" and the "abuse of" of sport. The underlying theoretical argument that can be made is as follows: Strong institutions (i.e., "forces" or "influences") govern society. Among those social institutions are:

145

(1) society's values (including created norms based on
    these values),
(2) the type of political state in vogue,
(3) the prevailing economic system,
(4) the religious beliefs present, etc.

To these longstanding institutions, I have over the years added such other influences as education, the communication media, science and technological advancement, concern for peace, *and now sport itself*. Of all of these, the ***values*** a society holds, and the accompanying norms developed on the basis of these values, form the strongest institution of all!

## Challenging the Role of Sport in Society

In "the Tiger Woods Saga", we find Tiger as a prominent figure in sport, a social institution whose influence has increased phenomenally. This development has become so vast that we may now ask whether it is accomplishing what it is presumably supposed to do. Is highly competitive sport as a social phenomenon doing more good than harm in society? The world seems to have accepted as fact that it is! Yet the world community does not really know whether this contention is true or not. Sport's expansion is permitted and encouraged almost without question in all quarters. "Sport is good for people, and more involvement with sport of almost any type--extreme sport, professional wrestling, missed martial arts, 'world cups'–even watching it regularly (!)--is better" seems to be the conventional wisdom. Witness, in addition, the billions of dollars that are being removed neatly out of tax revenues for the several Olympic enterprises perennially.

As I analyzed the "Tiger Woods Saga," I found it impossible to avoid a critique of commercialized sport as well. I believe that the development is now such that society should be striving to keep sport's drawbacks and/or excesses in check to the greatest possible extent. In recent decades we have witnessed the rise of sport throughout the land to the status of a fundamentalist religion. For example, we find sport being called upon to serve as a "redeemer of wayward youth," but--as it is occurring elsewhere—I believe it is also becoming a destroyer of certain fundamental values of individual and social life.

Wilcox, for example, in his empirical analysis, challenged "the widely held notion that sport can fulfill an important role in the development of national character." He stated: "the assumption that sport is conducive to the development of positive human values, or the 'building of character,' should be viewed more as a belief rather than as a fact." He concluded that sport did "provide some evidence to support a relationship between participation in sport and the ranking of human values" (1991, pp. 3, 17, 18, respectively).

Assuming Wilcox's view has reasonable validity, those involved in any way in the institution of sport--if they all together may be considered a collectivity--should contribute a quantity of redeeming social value to our North American culture, not to mention the overall world culture (i.e., a quantity of good leading to improved societal well-being). On the basis of this argument, the following two questions can be postulated for response by concerned agencies and individuals (e.g., federal governments, state and provincial officials, philosophers in the discipline and related professions):

(1) Can, does, or should a great (i.e., leading) nation produce great sport?

(2) With the world being threatened environmentally in a variety of ways, should we now be considering the "ecology" of sport as we are doing with other human activity? Both the beneficial and disadvantageous aspects of a particular sporting activity should be studied through the endeavors of scholars in various disciplines as well?

(3) If it is indeed the case that the guardian of the "functional satisfaction" resulting from sport is (a) the sports person, (b) the spectator, (c) the businessperson who gains monetarily, (d) the sport manager, and, in some instances, (e) educational administrators and their respective governing boards, then who in society should be in a position to be the most knowledgeable about the immediate objectives and long range aims of sport and related physical activity?

Answering these questions is a complex matter. First, as stated above, sport and related physical activity have become an extremely powerful social force in society. Secondly, if we grant that sport now has significant power in almost all of the world's developed cultures--a power indeed that appears to be growing--we should also recognize that any such social force affecting society is dangerous if perverted (e.g., through an excess of nationalism or commercialism). With this in mind, I am stating further that sport has somehow achieved such status as a powerful societal institution without an adequately defined underlying theory. Somehow, most countries seem to be proceeding generally on a typically unstated assumption that "sport is a good thing for society to encourage, and *more* sport is even better!" And yet, as explained above, the term "sport" exhibits radical ambiguity based on both everyday usage and dictionary definition. This obviously adds even more to the present problem and accompanying confusion.

This "radical ambiguity" about the role of sport takes us back to "the Tiger Woods Saga". Sport has now become a powerful social institution exerting influence for the betterment of society. Then, all of a sudden, a "sport hero" of the highest magnitude behaves himself in such a way that basic societal values are challenged. Hence, we now must ask ourselves: "Specifically what are *the* values that Tiger has forsaken that have occasioned this world-wide outburst of publicity"?

## "Socio-Instrumental" Values or "Moral" Values?

Examining this matter carefully, we may be surprised to learn that sport's contribution to human wellbeing is a highly complicated matter. On the one side, there are those who claim that sport contributes significantly to the development of what are regarded as the *socio-instrumental* values--that is, the values of teamwork, loyalty, self-sacrifice, aggressiveness, and perseverance consonant with prevailing corporate capitalism in democracy and in most other political systems as well. In the process of making this "contribution," however, we discover also that there is now a good deal of evidence that in the process of contributing to the "global ideal" of capitalism, democracy, and advancing technology, sport has developed an ideal that opposes the historical, fundamental *moral* values of honesty, fairness, good will, sportsmanship, and responsibility in the innumerable competitive experiences provided (Lumpkin, Stoll, and Beller, 1999).

Significant to this discussion are the results of investigations carried out by Hahm, Stoll, Beller, Rudd, and others in recent years. The Hahm-Beller Choice Inventory (HBVCI) has now been administered to athletes at different levels in a variety of venues. It demonstrates conclusively that athletes are increasingly *not* supporting what is considered "the moral ideal" in competition. As Stoll and Beller (1998) reported, for example, an athlete with moral character demonstrates the moral character traits of honesty, fair play, respect, and responsibility whether an official is present to enforce the rules or not. (Priest, Krause, and Beach substantiated this finding in 1999). They reported that changes over a four-year period in a college athlete's ethical value choices were consistent with other investigations. Their findings showed *decreases* in "sportsmanship orientation" and an *increase* in "professional" attitudes associated with sport bespeaking so-called "social" values..

Aha! We have now arrived at the nub of the matter! Alas for poor Tiger Woods... His plight is that he is "caught" right in the middle of this ongoing controversy about the presumed contribution of sport. No matter which way he turns, he is "out of step" with the claims for sport made by either group. His actions clash with those who say that sport contributes to *socio-instrumental* values. In addition, they also clash with those who argue that sport contributes to *moral* values. The perennial winner in golf, poor Tiger can't win now for losing! On the one hand he has confounded those who argue for "the social-values contribution", and–on the other hand–he has betrayed those who promote sport because it makes "a moral-values contribution". Hence, some of his advertisers are now deserting Tiger because his commercial value to them has been tarnished perhaps irrevocably. The gross stock value of his many sponsors has decreased appreciably since Tiger has been exposed. Concurrently, the sports *hero*, that staunch fellow presumably with all of those fine moral values, has betrayed his fans young and old because of his "nocturnal peregrinations." Woe is Tiger!

**Concluding Statement**

Even though dictionaries define *social* character similarly, many sport practitioners, including participants, coaches, parents, and officials, have gradually come to believe that character is defined properly by such values as self-sacrifice, teamwork, loyalty, and perseverance. The common expression in competitive sport is: "He or she showed character"--meaning "He/she 'hung in there' to the bitter end!" [or whatever...]. Rudd (1999) confirmed that coaches explained character as "work ethic and commitment." This coincides with what sport sociologists have found. Sage (1998. p. 614) explained: "Mottoes and slogans such as 'sports builds character' must be seen in the light of their ideological issues." In other words, competitive sport is structured by the nature of the society in which it occurs. This would appear to mean that over-commercialization, drug-taking, cheating, bribe-taking by officials, violence, etc. at all levels of sport are simply reflections of the culture in which we live.

Robert Osterhoudt (2010), one of the world's leading sport philosophers, offers a fundamental distinction to this troubling development as follows:

> it does seem to me as well that such social values as earnest
> effort, dedication, self-sacrifice, and the like are meaningfully talked

about in respect to sport and become defensible features of it *only if* they occur in the service of sport's inherent character as playful, competitive, and physical, not if they occur in the service of other forms of aim, such as commercial, nationalist, or military aim in particular. *The most fundamental distinction in all of this is thus the dividing of intrinsic and instrumental values, not the dividing of moral and social values.* (This is so because moral values, as described, serve *inherently*, thus becoming distinctly human ends.)

Where does all of this leave us today as we consider sport's presumed relationship with both *moral* character development and with *socio-instrumental* character development? Whatever your conclusion may be, Tiger Woods has been unexpectedly trapped in this "socio-instrumental" versus "moral" character vise that characterizes sport participation at the beginning of the 21st century. He tried to have it both ways. For his and his family's sake, let us hope that he will learn from this tragic experience—and that "the world" will "forgive his sins"…

**Example #5 (Corruption in Sport Internationally)**
**Corruption Followed as Cricket Grew in India**
(gleaned from a report by Jim Yardley
in WORLD, New Delhi, 2010 05 11)

In Chapter 8 of this volume, the plan is to demonstrate the kaleidoscopic nature of problems that are arising with the development of commercialized sport worldwide. An article written by Jim Yardley about possible graft in professional cricket in India surfaced in WORLD on May 11, 2010.

Yardley points out that allegations of graft in the India Premier League of cricket simply points out the extent to which corruption I still rampant in India.

The Indian Premier League has been established for only three years, and already business titans have managed to buy teams and make it all glamorous and sexy by the importation of Bollywood stars. The value of the league is reported to have risen to four billion dollars already. Evidently the commissioner of the League is under scrutiny by the authorities.

The league has tended to become a "symbol of a newly dynamic and confident India expanding its influence in the world. Nevertheless, after a series of allegations of financial irregularities, a minister of the government has resigned and the League's commissioner has been suspended. The result is that the happenings are pointing out that there is continuing corruption among India's "political and business elite."

The editor of *India today*, Aroon Purie, recently stated: "The great pity in India is that creations like the I.P.L. became a victim of their own success." He believes that the presence of so much money in activity inevitably leads to corruption/ Further, he implies that the sport of cricket may be confusing to the rest of the world outside of England, but somehow India has become obsessed with it.

All of this has government tax examiners to seize accounting records as they search for irregularities. Further, there is speculation that the I.P.L. commissioner has himself been able to amass much wealth through underhanded dealings. All of this presents difficulties as well for cricket board, a nongovernmental organization thst is somehow populated by a number of top politicians.

Historically, politicians have been overly involved in the sport with every state having a cricket association often headed by a prominent politician. This arrangement was obviously helpful to the sport's early development, but before long there were problems created by too great emphasis on commercialism including the introduction of cheerleaders and movie starts. Then a modified form of the game and its rules were created to conform to television time limits

Bollywood's stars began appearing in the stands at games. Soon a number of women began to show interest in the sport on television." Ramachandra Guha, a sport historian, felt that the League was being tailored to the middle class and to take attention awau from societal corruption and India's great inequality in its culture. In some ways India is doing well financially, but there are still 800,000 million people "far afield" from "the good life."

A variety of other investigations are occurring, also. However, somehow it seems that the "cricket situation" is unique by combining the best and worst of Indian capitalism.

**Example #6:** *(The Changing Scene*
*in Canadian Higher Education*
**Selective Response to the Document:**
**Queen's University Athletics and Recreation:**
**Charting a Course of Excellence.**
**by P. J. Galasso, Ph.D.**

Oct. 23, 2007

To Dr. Karen Hitchcock, Principal, Queen's University

cc. Chair, Board of Trustees; Chancellor; Rector; Associate Vice-Principal and Dean of Student Affairs; Director, School of Kinesiology and Health Studies; President, AMS; President, QUAA; Immediate Past-President, QUAA; Director of Athletics; Drs. Crawford and Deakin

I (P. J. Galasso) am responding because I am indebted to Queen's to such an extent that I could never repay it for what it did for me. I believe that I bring a broad and in-depth perspective to this issue.

> (**Note**: Some of my pertinent, related experiences are indicated at the end of this reaction to the document.)

I am responding because I see this approach as both damaging the experience of the student involved in inter-university sports and potentially interfering with his/her academic aspirations. I see it as a form of adulation of the scoreboard which will place undue pressures on the coaches and in turn on the students. So much attention could be placed on the inter-university programs that the sport clubs and recreation programs could be neglected.

**Comments/Questions Re Executive Summary:**

Breadth of opportunity means a wide number of inter-university sports as well as opportunities in recreation and fitness.

Excellence can also mean an overemphasis on winning with students being subjected to undue pressures from coaches intent upon retaining their positions, and thus potentially interfering with their academic aspirations.

152

The pursuit of excellence can mean money under the table to athletes and coaches. This could easily lead to use of drugs and other substances to enhance performance.

Will students be called upon to ignore injuries or downplay them?

Will trainers be under greater pressure to get players back into the game before they are ready?

Personal development of the students will take a back seat to being looked upon as a means to someone else's end.

Is this approach to excellence simply a means of satisfying "institutional ego"?

What will happen to teams that are dropped? Will they simply disappear or become sport clubs?

What will students whose teams are dropped, in later life after graduation, say to the personnel in Planned Giving when they come calling?

Raising the athletics and recreation fee could be viewed as a way of asking the student body to subsidize the athletic scholarships?

Is recommendation #14 a form of queue jumping?

Where do the numbers on a football team fit into the gender-equity picture? These numbers must be taken into account as individuals and not as a team.

Re Page 6: Queen's vision – Canada and nothing less.

The authors cite this as the basis for stating that nothing less than Canadian Championships are worthwhile as the ultimate goal of the inter-university program. This will lead us to overemphasis on winning. The scoreboard "über alles".

The last paragraph on this page alludes to benefits, but even here they talk about "getting connected" rather than referring to the values of individual growth and development under the tutelage of a well-rounded coach.

## What Winning Means and Will Lead to in the Proposal

Athletic scholarships (and where will the $ come from?), Higher student athletic fees,

Dogmatic adherence to NCCP status as basis for selecting coaches,

Canadian championships are the only ones that really count,

Coaches will be forced to spend more time recruiting than coaching,

Far fewer students will have an inter-university athletic experience,

Queen's will lose a great deal of its autonomy and educational values by designating itself as a farm team to various leagues, international bodies and competitions, etc.

and

Fundamentally, by placing the winning of Canadian championships as the most important basis for measuring success--as THE definition of excellence--the proposal slants dramatically its criteria for sport eligibility for candidacy to the inter-university status. This, plus the resultant, required coach selection and retention emphasis as well, will mean that the collective, student value-based experience fades into nonexistence. The student becomes an entertainer (i.e., a means to a different end). This is **elitism** at its worst. This is revealed in the box on page 18.

I could continue ad infinitum arguing with the stated and inherent premises of this document. I believe deep in my heart that the process has to be reinitiated with the experience of the student as the "number one" factor in deciding the major issues at hand. The experience of the student and the values they acquire--how they develop as human beings--is the most salient issue in formulating the basis of a program of interuniversity athletics including which teams are to be included in it. Everything else is secondary. Excellence will emerge through the appointment of topflight, experienced human beings designated as coaches who will bring out the best in the student by helping him/her to maximize their potential.

## Some Closing Remarks:

Drs. Crawford and Deakin have spent an enormous amount of time assembling their proposal. I respect the dedication that went into the effort. Sadly, at the fork in the road, they and I go in very different directions. We seem to be headed toward the "Big 10" U.S. model.

Dr. Earle F. Zeigler, in his paper, 'Where have they gone? (or How about a Canadian "Ivy League" in Inter-university sport?)', raises many issues that Canadian universities should take into account before taking the jump into what he terms "semiprofessional" sport. He identifies cheating, drugs, universities serving as international farm teams, and the unfairness of having students where academic standards are being maintained competing against athletes at less-demanding institutions. He concludes his paper with the following poignant statement: "At the university level, we have a sufficient number of problems while we strive to avoid shabbiness because of inadequate support. Permitting an increasing, unhealthy type of "athletic-scholarship mentality" to "creep" into university and college sport would eventually make us ridiculous and laughable to those who truly understand how it "ought to be." It's better to be proud and somewhat poorer financially, yet remain honorable and fair as we promote fine educational and recreational sport for all of our students." *Note*: Dr. Zeigler, a dual citizen, taught and coached at Yale, and was an administrator in physical education programs at Michigan and Illinois. He also was appointed to two terms as administrator at The University of Western Ontario, the latter as Dean of the newly structured Faculty of Physical Education.

Dr. Patrick J. Harrigan, sums up the situation in Canada in this statement taken from his paper given at the NASSH 2007 conference:

"Over the last half century, Canadian universities have suffered a series of financial crises that have threatened the very existence of its intercollegiate sports programs, sometimes regionally sometimes nationally. The first response was twofold. Internally universities introduced athletic or user fees. Nationally the CIAU sought sponsors to support intercollegiate championships in the late 60s. By the 1990s universities solicited alumni donations to save programs. Finally, both CIAU and universities elicited corporate sponsors to preserve intercollegiate teams. These problems have contributed to increased commercialization of major intercollegiate sport in Canada and threats to its traditions and amateur status. Dr. Harrigan expands upon the theme of commercialization of intercollegiate sport throughout his paper. Dr. Harrigan is the former head of the Department of History at the University of Waterloo.

The academic entrance requirements at Queen's, no doubt, have contributed significantly to the shortfall of Canadian championships. The recommendation that the entrance requirements be lowered for athletes does not sit well.

A code of ethics for those recruiting should be developed and monitored.

Coaches should be eligible for tenure.

Poor training and competition facilities need to be taken into account when deciding which sports should be dropped. Why build a hockey arena and drop hockey? Why build a field house and drop track and field? Where is the congruency?

Threat of discontinuance of a sport will harm recruiting.

Was Queen's pushed into the awarding of athletic scholarships or did it "jump"? If it jumped, the question is "Why"?

It would be beneficial if a major program on nutrition could be added to the fitness and wellness segment, something far beyond the Canada Food Rules and beyond obesity challenges as well. I would like to suggest that the work of Dr. Abram Hoffer, M.D., Ph.D. of Victoria, along with his cohorts in the field of orthomolecular medicine, be featured prominently in this segment.

Coaching is the heart of the program I would like to see implemented and augmented beyond what is now in existence. The healthy development of students in competitive situations would be quite beneficial. This is the ultimate basis for judgment, success, and excellence, not the scoreboard.

P. J. Galasso, Ph.D.

> **Note:** The following experiences are included (and listed *chronologically*) only to explain my early background and continuing interest in the subject at hand: (1) Canadian long jump champion; (2) AMS Athletic Stick and chair of Men's Intramural Council, Queen's University; (3) University head track and field and x-country Coach; (4) High school teacher and coach; (5) Queen's first director of athletics; (6) University intramural director; (7) President, Canadian Association for Health, Physical Education and Recreation; (8) Founding dean of Faculty of Human

Kinetics, University of Windsor; (9) taught ethics in sport and physical activity for 25 years; and (10) co-authored and edited a text in this area.

## Concluding Statement *(to Chapter 8)*

I confess to having just "scratched the surface" of the great number of serious problems facing sport at all levels (i.e., amateur, semi-professional, or professional). For example, the problem of substance-injection (infusion?) has become endemic to modern-day sport. Five days a week I receive an e-mail report from the Canadian Centre for Ethics in Sport that is performing such outstanding service to help the sport institution both within Canada and also worldwide. (See www.cces.ca) Day after day under such headings as "Doping and Sport," "Ethics and Sport," "Health and Physical Activity," and "Olympics," subscribers to this free service backed by an agency of the Canadian government are kept up to date on this devastating problem confronting sport worldwide at all levels.

As these words are being written, for example, a "Steroid Scandal rocks Waterloo" appeared in the Vancouver Sun (2010 06 15, C4). This article tells how the University has just suspended its intercollegiate football program for the year because nine members of the squad were potentially involved because of positive tests for steroids. This testing took place because another team member wad been arrested earlier and charged with drug possession and trafficking of steroids to his teammates,

Another area of concern is that of tracing the level of violence in contemporary sport and those activities being "invented" seemingly daily. For example, the wives of professional football players in America's National Football League have been organizing because of the drastic increase in early dementia appearing in the athletes (especially the linemen) due to head trauma "in the line of duty.".

Similarly, the longstanding "culture of violence" including the ready acceptance of violence in NHL hockey–*not Olympic hockey!*–draws the crowds, but promoters fail to take into consideration the present and future health and welfare of players.

Consider an extreme example: The instance in Iraq in 2008 when a soccer player was shot and killed just as he was to kick the "winning goal" in a match. Let's face it! Promoting the idea that winning is is the "one and only concern" of competitive sport should not be the main concern as we encourage children and youth to be involved.

Somehow (!), sport, designed originally to help youth and adults cope with ever more complex societal life with its accompanying conflict and turmoil, is itself ending up as one of the world major "blind spots." This has happened because of overemphasis and extreme commercialization that falls squarely into the lap of unbridled capitalism and onrushing technology.

What does all this mean? Simply put, it means that the determination of what constitutes "athletic success" is indeed a highly complex matter. The media give major space, of course, to professional sport and semiprofessional university sport. Administrators in colleges and universities where commercialism is under control must counter at every turn the efforts of uninformed people to relate success only to an individual's or a team's won-loss record, or to the amount of money taken in at the gate. Athletic success can and should have a relatively different meaning for those who make up the institution's internal and external environment.

What, then, should be considered success in football (or any sport for that matter)? Schools, colleges, and universities have too often been forced to consider the *extrinsic* results from sport competition. Now they should recognize that they also desperately need yardsticks to help them assess the *intrinsic* worth of the various aspects of their competitive sport programs. These aspects or characteristics can indeed be evaluated.

My recommendations regarding the more intrinsic characteristics of sport success are as follows:

*A high school, college, or university may claim athletic success if and only if the following occurs regularly at the following levels within your program:*

> 1. The Individual--you have success in football, for example, if the major objective in your program is whether your growth, maturity, skill, and fitness are improved as a result of the athletic experience.

> 2. The Team--you have success if an important objective in your program is with the quality of the competitive/cooperative experience, and whether there was sound improvement in the team's performance with a spirit of camaraderie and sportsmanship prevailing.

> 3. The Athletics Administrator--you have athletic success if the

recognized concern of the sport/athletic administrator of your institution is interpreting and carrying forward the philosophy and established policies and procedures of the institution so that an efficient and effective program of competitive sport results.

4. The Coach (and assistants)--you have athletic success if your concern as a coach in your program *demonstrates* that you are a dedicated professional educator who (1) possesses great respect for the
worth of the individual; (2) has an excellent knowledge and background in football; and (3) has the type of personality to inspire young men to achieve their potential within the demands of an educational environment.

5. The Game Officials--you have athletic success if your concern is to provide qualified game and contest officiating that is carried out by officials who have an understanding and appreciation of the educational institutions in the league or conference in which they are officiating. (This may be difficult to evaluate.)

6. The Educational Institution--you have football success if the concern in your program is that the president, vice-presidents, deans, professors, and students have a true understanding of the educational and non-commercial objectives of the institution's athletics program for boys and girls and young men men and women and base their judgment of athletic performance accordingly.

7. The Board of Trustees, Education, or Governors, etc.--you have athletic success if the concern in your program is that the administrators make every effort to educate you and other board members so that you will evaluate athletic performance fairly, and so that you will understand the strengths and weaknesses of the program in keeping with the institution's or agency's avowed educational philosophy and its ability to support that position.

8. The Local Community--you have athletic success if the concern in your program is to work as constructively as possible with the public so that members of the local community are fully informed as to the institution's competitive sport philosophy and can share in

the best possible realization of these broad educational goals.

9. The State or Provincial Legislature--you have athletic success if the concern of your state- or provincially supported institution is (a) to make every effort to ensure that the elected members of the legislature understand the institution's or agency's competitive sport policy; (b) that they have an opportunity for input into this policy's growth, development, and realization; and (c) that they be fully aware of the dangers of excess commercialism as it affects such a valuable medium for the achievement of a sound educational–recreational experience for our young people.

10. The Nation--you have athletic success if the concern in your program is to maintain the sport teams at all levels within the nation within an educational–recreational perspective so that citizens, including former participants and other supporters, may take pride in the overall achievement of the country's competitive sport program, while at the same time keeping well in mind the fact that regular, often excessive media publicity may well mean that undesirable influences are present and should possibly be curtailed.

The United States started going astray slowly but surely--notably with football--around the turn of the 20th century with its intercollegiate sport. Even President Teddy Roosevelt tried to straighten it out to no avail. Despite all of the efforts of the rules-governing bodies, this trend has increased to the point where by and large the "gate- receipt element" has continued as a highly important factor in the intercollegiate sport picture. And today, discouragingly, a heavy majority of Blacks in gate-receipt sports have not been completing their degree programs in four years at these "major" universities because of the demands of the program. Further, the effect of this unhealthy, commercialized development on high school sport has become most obvious as well.

Some may say that the 10 characteristics of athletic success presented above are hopelessly idealistic, and the claim could be made by the representatives of just about any school, college, or university, that their officials and coaches think they are approximating the ideal now. However, these educational institution in the United States especially are often not living up to the letter of their inadequate rules. *Further, the spirit of those statements hasn't a prayer of prevailing at this time.*

What does this mean ultimately? It tells us that something at the core is rotten and must somehow be rooted out. This is why improved evaluative techniques need to be developed, enforced, and maintained by national sports-governing bodies. And, to prevent ever-present undue pressures by alumni and businesspeople, the federal government—as they did with the implementation of Title 9 for girls' and women's sport—may itself have to get involved to overcome such educational deficiency.

Some will argue that commercialism and excessive media attention do not necessarily mean that a program can't be educationally sound. Conceivably this could be true, but much of the experience in the United States has shown that such a beneficial outcome is highly unlikely. It has certainly now become a debatable question whether—under the prevailing conditions operative in all save "Ivy League-type institutions"—sport does more harm than good.

It is interesting to note that the large majority of other countries haven't fallen prey to many of the same influences that have made helpless laughing stocks of many dignified, beleaguered, well- intentioned, yet overwhelmed university and college presidents in the United States. (*This is not to say that overemphasis and commercialism has not affected competitive sport I the public sector in these countries.*) These American administrators tried to take control, but they have consistently been shunted aside. If they as individual presidents become too obstreperous, for example, they will inevitably be forced to the sidelines. Generally speaking, "The tail is wagging the dog" in the United States. Citizens in other lands should struggle to "keep their dog both clear- headed and amateur in fact and in spirit--with all four legs solidly beneath him!"

# Chapter 9
## Creating Positive Values Through Developmental Physical Activity

Despite this steady increase in competitive sport offerings, just about all of us would admit readily that there should always be more to life than sport. We are quick to criticize the young person who doesn't appear to be rounding into normal maturity. At a certain age we typically expect youth to become interested in the opposite sex--an unrealistic expectation for all today--and develop heterosexual social recreational interests.

We like to think also that young people are developing in other areas of recreational interest–in communicative interests such as conversation and discussion, as well as in writing and in learning interests that indicate a desire to know more about many aspects of the world that interest them. This development should further extend to creative and aesthetic interests where the opportunity is afforded to create beauty according to individual appreciation of what constitutes artistic expression of form, color, sound, or movement.

However, I agree that we can't state absolutely or precisely that such-and-such a program *should* be followed. Living one's life will always be (we hope) an art rather than a science. Nevertheless, people who are maturing should proceed basically on the best available theory based on scientific findings. The opinions of educators, of medical scientists, and of social scientists point in a similar direction, of course, but often this is still based on inadequate evidence.

*Nevertheless, I believe strongly that physical activity education (including athletics and related health instruction), broadly interpreted and experienced under wise educational or recreational conditions, can serve humankind as a worthwhile social institution contributing vitally to the well being, ongoing health, and longevity of humankind.*

## This Disoriented Field Involving Human Physical Activity Should Have a Mission?

Despite my italicized statement immediately above, this message is simply not getting across to the population in advanced countries to such an extent that it is being implemented to the right degree! Every year the *Quest journal* devotes one issue to report the proceedings of the previous year's annual meeting of the American Academy of Kinesiology and Physical Education. The 2006 theme of the AAKPE was "Kinesiology: Defining the Academic Core of Our Discipline."

Michael Wade, director the School of Kinesiology at the University of Minnesota, was asked to be the conference summarizer. His "Quo Vadis Kinesiology?" analysis raised some excellent, pointed questions about the essence of the program held. Accepting the fact that the field ("we" referring to members of the Academy "have at least tentatively decided to call itself kinesiology," Wade continued with a number of insightful reactions that pointed out our field's highly disturbing lack of orientation that is characterized by the absence of a clear statement of mission.

> (Note: Wade, M. (2007) "Quo Vadis Kinesiology?" In *Quest*, 59, 1, pp. 170-173.)

I immediately wrote him expressing some of the thoughts below. For example, it seemed that we had some agreement as to the "rudderlessness" of the Academy and the entire field itself. As I read the proceedings, I was greatly discouraged by the program planning and subsequent proceedings of this disparate group. The individual statements of the invited speakers at this meeting were generally excellent. However, it was the central focus that was so woefully inadequate!

These men and women are the self-proclaimed 100 "top, active scholars and scientists" of "kinesiology and physical education" in the USA! This is the scholarly group that deliberately separated itself in the early 1990s from the founding professional society, the one that spawned us all! (The AAHPERD was originally the Association for the Advancement of Physical Education in 1885).

> (Note: At this point I should explain my intense interest in the topic] because I was inducted as a Fellow in the [then] Academy of Physical Education in 1966 and subsequently was elected president. Finally, I received its highest recognition: the Hetherington Award.)

Now, concluding my 70th active year in the field that has been searching for a "consensual name" for more than a a century, I admit that I too thought that the question had been resolved. I can remember C. H. McCloy (arguably the top "physical educator/scientist" of the first half of the 20th century) saying: "To change the name away from *physical education* now would be akin to rolling back Niagara Falls." (Interestingly, this interesting predictions seem to has on occasion been accomplished

I am trying hard, also, not to become "un ancien". (Since the turn of the 21st century, some sixteen books, other monographs, and articles of mine have been published.) The AAKPE's "progress" or "status"–admittedly of long standing and significant stature in this field–is in a way something like that of the more recent International Association for Sport Philosophy, another group of which I was president also in an "earlier life." The public doesn't know that the IAPS exists; the field of education doesn't know it exists; and physical activity educators and coaches worldwide don't know (or care!) that it's there either. Interestingly, the people from different "specialties" within each of these societies don't typically "speak" to each other during the year as well. Hence, I must ask: Whom have I missed that members of both societies are not speaking to?

My question is simply this: If these groups do not relate strongly to the public, to education, and to the established field of practitioners closest to the discipline they represent, what good are they? (Oh yes, for the moment I forgot. Their societal publications are vital for individuals' on-the-job promotion and for obtaining funds to attend conferences!) In semi-retirement at age 90, I will continue--for a while, I hope--to write for those in the field concerned about "physical activity education in exercise, sport, dance, and physical recreation–accompanied by related health education–for normal, accelerated, special people of all ages ".

We–as members of a quasi-discipline, quasi-profession–want this for everybody. In addition, we can get knowledge and assistance for the fulfillment of our mission by turning to all of the humanities, the social science, and the natural sciences--as well as a variety of professions and working specifically with them. For example, I ask, what knowledge is "out there" in the subject of geography that can further healthful physical activity? Or in anthropology? Or kinanthropometry?

Fundamentally, as I said in an e-book: "As professionals we don't know what we don't know because the burgeoning knowledge component of our various sub disciplinary and sub-professional components has gotten away from any one person!" Frankly, this is where our professional associations worldwide can and should be helping practitioners by providing "evolving ordered generalizations" of scientific and scholarly findings about developmental physical activity.

Frankly, and bluntly, I can come to no other conclusion other than that a solid segment of the people in our field at the university level are undoubtedly candidates for recognition as the most disoriented group of scientists and scholars in existence. I'm sure there are other disoriented groups "out there" as well that I'm not aware of. These are people who have what the late Paul Hunsicker of our field (Michigan, Ann Arbor) used to call "tunnel vision."

We in this field *within education* have not been given the necessary support to work at all levels within the field of education (children, teens, adults, etc.) In addition, the field was not able to flourish or develop in society at large to work with adults, "middle-agers," and seniors. ***YET THE DIRE NEED FOR REGULAR PLANNED PHYSICAL ACTIVITY (Exercise!) FOR ALL THROUGHOUT THEIR LIVES IS SO OBVIOUS!***

What did happen? It has now become a little bit like what Jimmy Durante, the late comedian, used to say: "Everybody's trying to get into the act!" A cacophony of "other voices" have entered the picture to fill the vacuum! Even my *Mayo Clinic Health Letters* includes sound physical activity education procedures written by presumably unqualified medical person because there is no author attribution)! Interestingly, there isn't a week that goes by without some new study pointing out that regular physical activity can cure or improve "this or that" in people's lives or lengthen their lives.

In addition, I am forced to ask further: What is going on here? How many of these graduates in the discipline of kinesiology (i.e., the study of movement literally) will be helping people in society to live better lives based on their qualifications as "movement analysts"? I'm certain that some will, but who knows about it? Where is the proof that these graduates of kinesiology programs are helping people of all ages to analyze movement kinematically (much less understand such movement **KINETICALLY**)? Shouldn't that--by definition!--be their function based on this Greek nomenclature?

Further, I would like to see the rationalization for the positions these graduates are engaged in. Where are they? What are they doing? Do we really know? A small percentage does go to the units of professional education on campuses to become teachers in a system where their efforts will continue to be downgraded. Why downgraded? Because **WE** in the field evidently haven't "made our case" strongly enough. Any statement of the field of physical activity education's mission should proclaim our hope that all people **WORLDWIDE,** people of all ages and conditions actively will be involved with satisfaction in healthful and joyful physical activity.

**Based on Established Principles,
We Should Guarantee the Best Type
Of Developmental Physical Activity To Youth**

*Physical Activity Education's
Fourteen (14) "Principal Principles"*

Principle 1: The "Reversibility Principle". The first principle affirms that cardio-vascular conditioning is inherently reversible in the human body;

Principle 2: The "Overload Principle". The second principle states that a muscle or muscle group must be taxed beyond that to which it is accustomed, or it won't develop;

Principle 3: The "Flexibility Principle". This principle indicates that a human must put the body's various joints through the range of motion for which they are intended. Inactive joints become increasingly inflexible until immobility sets in;

Principle 4: The "Bone Density Principle". This principle asserts that developmental physical activity throughout life helps significantly to maintain the density of a human's bones;

Principle 5: The "Gravity Principle". This principle explains that maintaining muscle-group strength throughout life, while standing or sitting, helps the human fight against the force of gravity that is working continually to break down the body's structure;

Principle 6: The "Relaxation Principle". Principle 6 states that the skill of relaxation is one that people must acquire in today's increasingly complex world;

Principle 7: The "Aesthetic Principle". This principle explains that a person has either an innate or culturally determined need to "look good" to himself/herself and to others;

Principle 8: The "Integration Principle". Principle 8 demonstrates that developmental physical activity is an important means whereby the individual can "fully involved" as a living organism. By their very nature, physical activities in exercise, sport, play, and expressive movement demand full attention from the organism--often in the face of opposition-- and therefore involve complete psycho-physical integration;

Principle 9: The "Integrity Principle". The principle of integrity implies that a completely integrated psycho-physical activity should correspond **ETHICALLY** with the avowed ideals and standards of society.(Thus, the "integrity principle" goes hand in hand with desirable integration of the human's various aspects [so-called unity of body and mind in the organism explained in Principle 8 immediately above]};

Principle 10: The "Priority of the Person Principle". Principle 10 affirms that any physical activity in sport, play, and exercise sponsored through public or private agencies should be conducted in such a way that the welfare of the individual comes first (i.e., sport must serve as a "social servant");

Principle 11: The "Live Life to Its Fullest Principle". This principle explains that, viewed in one sense, human movement is what distinguishes the individual from the rock on the ground. Unless the body is moved with reasonable vigor according to principles 1-6 above, it will not serve a person best throughout life;

Principle 12: The "Fun and Pleasure Principle". Principle 12 states that the human is normally a "seeker of fun and pleasure," and that a great deal of the opportunity for such enjoyment can be derived from full, active bodily movement; and

Principle 13: The "Longevity Principle". This recently conceived principle affirms the possibility that regular developmental physical activity throughout life can help a person live longer (Zeigler, 1994).

Principle 14: The "Physical Fitness & Learning–Correlation Principle" affirms that evidence accumulating is showing a positive relationship between physical fitness and what is termed as academic achievement.

## The Professional Task Ahead

What, then, is the professional task ahead? First, we should truly understand why we have chosen this profession as we rededicate ourselves anew to the study and dissemination of knowledge, competencies, and skills in developmental physical activity in sport, exercise, and related expressive movement. Concurrently, of course, we need to determine exactly what it is that we are professing.

Second, as either professional practitioners or instructors involved in professional preparation, we should search for young people of high quality in all the attributes needed for success in the field. Then we should follow through to help them develop lifelong commitments so that our profession can achieve its democratically agreed-upon goals. We should also prepare young people to serve in the many alternative careers in sport, exercise, dance, and recreational play that are becoming increasingly available in our society.

Third, we must place *quality* as the first priority of our professional endeavors. Our personal involvement and specialization should include a high level of competency and skill under girded by solid knowledge about the profession. It can be argued that our professional task is as important as any in society. Thus, the present is no time for indecision, half-hearted commitment, imprecise knowledge, and general unwillingness to stand up and be counted in debate with colleagues within our field and in allied professions and related disciplines, not to mention the public.

Fourth, the obligation is ours. If we hope to reach our potential, we must sharpen our focus and improve the quality of our professional effort. Only in this way will we be able to guide the modification process that the profession is currently undergoing toward the achievement of our highest professional goals. This is the time, right now, to employ exercise, sport, dance, and play to make our reality more healthful, more pleasant, more vital, and more life enriching. By "living fully in one's body," behavioral science men and women will be adapting and shaping this phase of reality to their own ends.

Finally, such improvement will not come easily; it can only come through the efforts of professional people making quality decisions, through the motivation of people to change their sedentary lifestyles, and through our professional assistance in guiding people as they strive to fulfill such motivation in their movement patterns. Our missions in the years ahead is to place this special quality in all of our professional endeavor.

## What Should The Field of Developmental Physical Activity Do in the 21st Century?

What should the field of developmental physical activity do--perhaps what *must* we do--to ensure that it will move more decisively and rapidly in the direction of what might be called status *within* education and recognized status as a profession in society at large? Granting that the various social forces will impact upon us, what can we do collectively in the years immediately ahead? These positive steps should be actions that will effect a workable consolidation of purposeful accomplishments on the part of those men and women who have a concern for the future of developmental physical activity as a valuable component of human life from birth to death. The following represent a number of categories joined with action principles that are related insofar as possible to the "modifications" that have been taking place in our field. We should seek a North American consensus on the steps spelled out below. Then we, as dedicated professional educators, should take as rapid and strong action as we can muster through our professional associations in America and Canada. These recommended steps are as follows:

*A Sharper Image.*  Because in the past the field of physical education has tried to be "all things to all people," and presently doesn't know exactly what it does stand for, we should now sharpen our image and improve the quality of our efforts by focusing primarily on developmental physical activity--specifically, human motor performance in sport, exercise, and related expressive movement. As we sharpen our image, we should make a strong effort to cooperate with those who are working in the private agency and commercial sectors by helping them to get organized under a *single* national association with related state and/or provincial entities. This implies further that we will extend our efforts to promote the finest type of developmental physical activity for people of all ages whether they be members of what are considered to be "normal, accelerated, or special" populations.

*Our Field's Name.*  Because all sorts of name changes have been implemented (a) to explain either what people think we are doing or should be doing, or (b) to camouflage the presumed "unsavory" connotation of the term "physical education" that evidently conjures up the notion of a "dumb jock" working with the lesser part of a tri-partite human body, we should continue to focus primarily on *developmental physical activity* as defined immediately above while moving toward an acceptable working term for our profession.  In so doing, we should keep in mind the field's bifurcated nature in that it has both theoretical and practical (or disciplinary and professional) aspects. At the moment we are called sport and physical education or physical activity and recreation (NASPE or AAPAR, respectively) within the Alliance (AAHPERD) professionally and physical and health education in a significant number of elementary and secondary schools in Canada (PHE Canada). A desirable name for our under girding discipline would be *developmental physical activity*, and we could delineate this by our inclusion of exercise, sport, and expressive movement. (As this book is being written, the terms "kinesiology" and "human kinetics" (from the Greek word *kinesis* are looming ever larger in both the United States and Canada as a name for the undergraduate degree program in our field. However, it is most difficult to see this word catching on in the public schools.)

*A Tenable Body of Knowledge.* Inasmuch as various social forces and professional concerns have placed us in a position where we don't know where or what our body of knowledge is, we will strongly support the idea of disciplinary definition and the continuing development of *a body of knowledge* based on such a consensual definition. From this must come a merging of tenable scientific theory in keeping with societal values and computer technology so that we will gradually, steadily, and increasingly provide our members with the knowledge that they need to perform as top-flight professionals. As professionals we simply must possess the requisite knowledge, competencies, and skills necessary to provide developmental physical activity services of a high quality to the public both within education and also in society at large.

*Our Own Professional Association.* Inasmuch as there is insufficient support of our own professional association for a variety of reasons, we need to develop voluntary and mandatory mechanisms that relate membership in **one** *professional* organization both directly and indirectly to stature within the field. We simply must now commit ourselves to work tirelessly and continually to promote the welfare of professional practitioners who are serving the public in the educational system and also in the larger society. Incidentally, it may be necessary to exert any available pressures to encourage people to give first priority to our own scholarly and professional groups (as opposed to those of related disciplines and/or allied professions). The logic behind this dictum is that our own survival comes first for us!

*Professional Licensing.* Although most teachers/coaches in the schools, colleges, and universities are seemingly protected indefinitely by the shelter of the all-embracing teaching profession, we should now move rapidly and strongly to seek official recognition of our endeavors in public, semi-public, and private agency work and in commercial organizations relating to developmental physical activity *through professional licensing at the state or provincial level.* Further, we should encourage individuals to apply for voluntary registration as qualified practitioners at the federal level in both the United States and Canada.

*Harmony Within The Field.* Because an unacceptable series of gaps and misunderstandings has developed among those in our field concerned primarily with the bio-scientific aspects of human motor performance, those concerned with the social-science and humanities aspects, those concerned with the general education of all students, those concerned with the professional preparation of physical activity educators/coaches, and those connected with the professional preparation of sport managers–all at the college or university level–we will strive to work for *a greater balance and improved understanding* among these essential entities within the profession.

*Harmony Among The Allied "Professions".* Keeping in mind that the original field of physical education has spawned a number of allied "professions" down through the years of the 20th century, *we should strive to comprehend what they claim that they do professionally, and where there may be a possible overlap with what we claim that we do.* Where disagreements prevail, they should be ironed out to the greatest extent possible at the national level within the Alliance (AAHPERD) in the United States and within Physical & Health Education Canada (PHE Canada).

*The Relationship With Intercollegiate Athletics/Sport.* An ever-larger wedge has been driven between units of physical education and interscholastic and intercollegiate athletics in educational institutions where gate receipts are a strong and basic factor. Such a rift serves no good purpose and is counter to the best interests of both groups. *Developmental physical activity available through the services of physical activity educators should remain separate from varsity sport in those universities where the promotion of highly organized, often commercialized athletics exists (e.g., NCAA Division I and II institutions).. However, we must work for greater understanding and harmony with those people who are primarily interested in this enterprise.* At the same time it is imperative that we do all in our power to maintain athletics in a sound educational perspective within our schools, colleges, and universities.

*The Relationship with Intramurals and Recreational Sports.* Intramurals and recreational sports is in a transitional state at present in that it has proved that it is "here to stay" at the college and university level. Nevertheless, intramurals hasn't really taken hold yet, generally speaking, as a program of after-school sport experiences at the high school level, despite the fact that it has a great deal to offer the large majority of "normal" and "special-needs" students in what may truly be called *educational* sport. Everything considered, I believe (1) that--both philosophically and practically--intramurals and recreational sports ought to remain within the sphere of the physical activity education field; (2) that it is impractical and inadvisable to attempt to subsume all non-curricular activities on campus under one department or division; and (3) that departments and divisions of physical activity education ought to work for consensus on the idea that *intramurals and recreational sports are co-curricular in nature* and deserve regular funding as laboratory experience in the same manner that general education course experiences in physical activity education receives its funding for instructional purposes.

*Guaranteeing Equal Opportunity.* Because "life, liberty, and the pursuit of happiness" are guaranteed to all in North American society. as a profession we should move positively and strongly to see to it that *equal opportunity* is indeed provided to the greatest possible extent to women, to minority groups, and to special populations (e.g., the handicapped) as they seek to improve the quality of their lives through the finest type of experience in the many activities of our field.

*Holding High the Physical Activity Education (including Sport) Identity.* In addition to the development of the allied professions (e.g., school health education) in the second quarter of the twentieth century, we witnessed the advent of a disciplinary thrust in the 1960s that was followed by a splintering of many of the various "knowledge components" and subsequent formation of many different societies. These developments have undoubtedly weakened the field of (sport and) physical education as it is now called within the NASPE and physical activity and recreation within the AAPAR. Thus, it is now more important than ever that we *hold high the physical activity education identity* as we continue to promote vigorously the scholarly academies that have been formed within the AAHPERD (and the similar scholarly interest groups [SIGS] with PHE Canada). Additionally we should re-affirm and delineate even more carefully our relationship with our allied professions.

*Applying a Competency Approach.* Whereas the failures and inconsistencies of the established educational process have become increasingly apparent, *we will as a field within the education profession and a profession in society at large explore the educational possibilities of a competency approach* as it might apply to general education, to professional preparation, and to all aspects of our professional endeavor in public, semi-public, private, and commercial agency endeavors

*Managing the Enterprise.* All professionals in the unique field of physical activity education (including sport) are managers--but to varying degrees. The "one course in administration" approach with no laboratory or internship experience of earlier times is simply not sufficient for the future. There is an urgent need to apply a competency approach in the preparation (as well as in the continuing education) of those who will serve as managers either within educational circles or elsewhere in the society at large.

*Ethics and Morality in Physical Activity Education (and Educational/Recreational Sport).* In the course of the development of the best professions, the various, embryonic professional groups have gradually become conscious of the need for a set of professional ethics--that is, a set of professional *obligations* that are established as *norms* for practitioners in good standing to follow. Our profession needs both a creed and a detailed code of ethics right now as we move ahead in our development. Such a move is important because, generally speaking, ethical confusion prevails in North American society. Development of a sound code of ethics, combined with steady improvement in the three essentials of a fine profession (i.e., an extensive period of training, a significant intellectual component that must be mastered before the profession is practiced, and a recognition by society that the trained person can provide a basic, important service to its citizens) would relatively soon place us in a much firmer position to claim that we are indeed members of a fine profession. (Zeigler, 2007).

*Reunifying the Field's Integral Elements.* Because there now appears to be reasonable agreement that what is now called the field of sport and physical education (within NASPE) and physical activity and recreation (within AAPAR), *we will is concerned primarily with developmental physical activity as manifested in human motor performance in sport, exercise, and related expressive movement. In addition, we will now work for the reunification of those elements of our profession that should be uniquely ours within our disciplinary definition of developmental physical activity.*

*Cross-Cultural Comparison and International Understanding.* We have done reasonably well in the area of international relations within the Western world due to the solid efforts of many dedicated people over a considerable period of time, but at present we need to redouble our efforts to make cross-cultural comparisons of physical activity education (including educational/recreational sport) while reaching out for international understanding and cooperation in both the Western and Eastern blocs. Much greater understanding on the part of all of the concepts of 'communication,' 'diversity,' and 'cooperation' is required for the creation of a better life for all in a *peaceful* world. Our profession can contribute significantly toward this long-range objective.

*Permanency and Change.* Inasmuch as the "principal principles" espoused for physical education in the early 1950s by the late Arthur Steinhaus of George Williams College have now been extended from four to fourteen, all still apply most aptly to our professional endeavors, *we will continue to emphasize that which is timeless in our work, while at the same time accepting the inevitability of certain societal change.*

*Improving the Quality and Length of Life.* Since our field is **unique** within education and in society, and since fine living and professional success involve so much more than the important verbal and mathematical skills, we will emphasize strongly that education is a lifelong enterprise. Further, we will stress that *the quality*

173

*and length of life can be improved significantly through the achievement of an acceptable degree of kinetic awareness and through heightened experiences in exercise, sport, and related expressive movement.*

*Reasserting Our "Will to Win".* Although the developments of the past 30 years have undoubtedly created an uneasiness within the profession, and have raised doubts on the part of some as to our possession of a "will to win" through the achievement of the highest type of professional status, *we pledge ourselves to make still greater efforts to become vibrant and stirring through absolute dedication and commitment in our professional endeavors.* Ours is a high calling as we seek to improve the quality of life for all through the finest type of developmental physical activity in sport, exercise, and related expressive movement.

# Chapter 10
# Fostering Physical Activity Values
# in the World of the Future

This is the final chapter of a book titled The Use and Abuse of Human Physical Activity. Keeping in mind the titles of almost every individual chapter to this point, I'm tempted to offer a "groaner" that "I hope you have found this to be a "value-able" experience." However, I won't be so crass as to suggest that such has been the case…

Nevertheless, if you have "stayed with me to the bitter end," I think you may agree that your values, my values, our values, the world's values are literally "what it's all about"! However, as I have tried to explain, there is so much confusion about the subject of values at all levels, and that is what is so discouraging. Yet, as perhaps you appreciate a bit more now, the fact that there is confusion occurs because of the complexity of the topic. Whatever, in this final chapter I will attempt to summarize briefly what we have covered in the same chronological order followed in the nine preceding chapters.

## The "What Are Humans?" Discussion

Recall that I did not go back to the very beginning of the universe and seek to explain its beginning and almost inconceivable enormity. Instead I asked you to "google" "The Universe" and then watch *the 10-minute video* that typically appears on the first page of items appearing on your screen.

I did, however, ask you to distinguish what has often been called "the adventure of civilization" while appreciating that the beginnings of the first civilization on Earth was only about 10,000 tears ago, Then I outlined the ways that humans learned to acquire knowledge (e.g., sensing) along with the four "historical revolutions" that have occurred in the development of the world's "communication capability" (e.g., writing),

Next I delineated the various "historical images" that have been created to describe what the essence of the individual is as he/she sought to cope with the surrounding environment (e.g., the human as a "rational animal"). Following this, I explained the seven rival theories about human nature as postulated by the insightful work of Leslie Stevenson (1987). Each of these prognostications was saying in essence: This is "the hand that humans have been dealt," and "this is how they can best react to it what such a finding is telling them" The Christian view of the human, for example, is that the nature of man is characterized as a creature made in the image of God and is destined to have control of the rest of God's creation.

A starkly different view of the human was offered by Konrad Lorenz's "innate aggression" theory about human nature. He argued that the happenings of early childhood are basic to a person's subsequent philosophical and later scientific development. His assumption was that the instinctual behavior patterns of a particular species occurred as a result of the individual's genes evolving down through the ages. Hence it is easy to understand why Darwin's *Origin of Species* (1859) caused such a furor when the human's evolution through so-called natural selection was propounded. "The world" has not been the same since this contradiction of Christian doctrine.

To this point we knew that we were organisms, living creatures, who have reached a stage of development where we "know that something has happened, is continuing to happen, and will evidently continue to happen." However, underlying my entire analysis I stated that I was searching for the answers to *two historical questions*: First, did humans in earlier times, equipped with their coalescing genes and evolving *memes*, enjoy to any significant degree what discerning people today might define as "quality living?" Second, I wondered whether earlier humans had any opportunity for freely chosen, beneficial physical activity in sport, exercise, play, and dance that was of sufficient quality and quantity to contribute to the quality of life.

Of course, I appreciated that asking a question about the quality of life in earlier times was doubly difficult, of course, because we appreciate that present-day humans can't be both judge and jury in such a debate. On what basis can we decide, for example, whether any social progress has indeed been made such that would permit resolution of such a concept as "quality living" including a modicum of "ideal sport competition" or "purposeful physical activity and related health education."?

There has been progression, of course, but how can we assume that change is indeed progress? It may be acceptable as a human criterion of progress to say that we are coming closer to approximating the good and the solid accomplishments that we think humans should have achieved both including what might be termed "the finest type" of sport competition

One realizes immediately, also, that any assessment of the quality of life in prerecorded history, including the possible role of sport in that experience, must be a dubious evaluation at best. However, I was intrigued by the work of Herbert Muller who has written so insightfully about the struggle for freedom in human history. I was impressed, also, by his belief that recorded history has displayed a "tragic sense" of life. Whereas the philosopher Hobbes (1588-1679) stated in his *De Homine* that very early humans existed in an anarchically individualistic state of nature in which life was "solitary, poor, nasty, brutish, and short," Muller (1961) argued in rebuttal that it "might have been poor and short enough, but that it was never solitary or simply brutish" (p. 6).

Accordingly, Muller's approach to history is "in the spirit of the great tragic poets, a spirit of reverence and or irony, and is based on the assumption that the tragic sense of life is not only the profoundest but the most pertinent for an understanding of both past and present" (1952, p. vii). The rationalization for his "tragic" view is simply that the drama of human history has truly been characterized by high tragedy in the Aristotelian sense. As he states, "All the mighty civilizations of the past have fallen, because of tragic flaws; as we are enthralled by any Golden Age we must always add that it did not last, it did not do" (p. vii).

This made me wonder whether the 20th century of the modern era might turn out to be the Golden Age of America. This may be true because so many misgivings are developing about former blind optimism concerning history's malleability and compatibility in keeping with American ideals. As Heilbroner (1960) explained in his 'future as history' concept, America's still-prevalent belief in a personal "deity of history" may be short-lived in the 21st century. Arguing that technological, political, and economic forces are "bringing about a closing of our historic future," he emphasized the need to search for a greatly improved "common denominator of values" (p. 178).

However, all of this could be an oversimplification, because the concept of 'civilization' is literally a relative newcomer on the world scene. At present we can never forget for a moment that previous human civilizations were not miraculously saved! Literally, not one has made it! Thus, "Man errs, but strive he must," admonished Goethe, and we as world citizens today dare not forget that dictum.

## What Are the Values Held by Humans?

Recall that axiology (the study of values) is the fourth subdivision of the discipline of philosophy and is (presumably!) the end result of philosophizing. The individual should strive to develop a system of values reasonably consistent with his or her beliefs in the other three subdivisions as well: metaphysics (or inquiry about the nature of reality); epistemology (or the study of knowledge acquisition); and logic (or the exact relating of ideas).

Values are principles or standards of behavior that people consider to be important or beneficial. They are basic and are an integral part of every culture. A person is a member of a culture and typically holds beliefs and assumptions about it and the world in which it functions.

The values people hold convey to others what is good and important in their lives. Accordingly, the defensible ethical decisions people make require a wise choice of values. However, even though humankind has won a recognizable semblance of victory over what is often a harsh physical environment, it is true that many people have not been able to remove much of the social insecurity that plagues their lives.

In addition, there is still no non-controversial foundation on which the entire structure of ethics can be built. Hence, as life becomes ever more complex in the early 21st century, there are at least *eight* major ethical routes to decision-making about values extant in what we call the Western world (Graham, 2004).

A basic question arises: Are values objective or subjective–that is, do values exist whether a person is present to realize them or not? Or is it merely people who ascribe value to the various relationships they have with others--and possibly also with their physical environment? In addition, if a value exists in and for itself, it is said to be an *intrinsic* value. One that serves as a means to an end, however, has become known as an *instrumental* or extrinsic value.

In the past, moral philosophers offered general guidance as to what to do, what to seek, and how to treat others--injunctions that we should be fully aware of even today. As a rule, however, philosophers have not tried to preach to their adherents in the same way that theologians have felt constrained to do. The earlier moral philosophers did, however, offer practical advice that included a great variety of pronouncements about what was good and bad, or right and wrong in human life.

Today it makes good sense that, with problems, conflicts and strife existing at all levels, a person should strive to get to the heart of this vital matter for the sake of his or her future. Unfortunately, the child and adolescent in what we call modern society are missing out almost completely on a sound "experiential" introduction to ethics. This has created what may be called an "ethical decision-making dilemma." Frankly, it is a *crisis* and represents a condemnation of present society!

The question is "What to do about this lack?" Where can one go from almost "inherent confusion" that exists in so many lives? The strategy being proposed here for improving this situation is that people should (1) list what they believe our values are in light of the changing times. Then—possibly in discussion with those who are closest to them—they should (2) rearrange and restate them in some type of graduated or hierarchical order.

Thereafter, finally, they will (3) need to assess more carefully--on a regular basis--whether they are living up to those values they have chosen, the values they so often glibly espouse whenever the occasion arises. This bold assertion makes good sense whether reference is being made to what takes place with a person and his or her family in the home, the school, the church, or in the everyday world.

## The Value/Ethics Relationship

As I explained earlier, in the discipline of philosophy, the term "value" is equivalent to the concepts of "worth" and "goodness". It is helpful, however, to draw a distinction between two kinds of value: (1) *intrinsic* value = human experience good or valuable in itself, an end for its own sake, and (2) *extrinsic* value = an experience about goodness or value similarly, while serving as a means to achieve some purpose or material gain.

Ethics is termed a *speculative* subdivision of philosophy that treats the question of values. (Axiology is the technical name for the actual study of values.) It has to do with morality, conduct, good, evil, and the ultimate objectives of life. As it has developed, there was an ongoing need for people to define values still further in human life. So now there are specialized philosophies of religion, education, art, and even of sport and physical activity education.

After the ancient Greeks, ethical thought was oriented more to practice than to theory. Also, the meanings of ethical terms and concepts did not change appreciably until marked social change occurred in the 16th and 17th centuries. At that point it was argued for the first time that ethics should be contrasted with science because the latter was presumably ethically neutral (i.e., value free).

Thereafter, in the Western world at least, a continuing struggle began between advocates of philosophical utilitarianism and those espousing idealism (i.e., the attempt to distinguish between naturalistic ethics and so-called moral law prescribed by some power greater than humans). This struggle has continued to the present day with no firm evidence that it will abate in the near future.

## A Persistent Problem for Humankind: Value Choice

Through the history of humankind, value choice became a persistent problem. If it is accepted that the values held by people in any particular era are so important, it holds also that the determination of "what is important" has been a "persistent problem" historically for humankind. If an individual or group sought to deviate from what the majority in a society felt about what was important or necessary, a crossroad or crisis in life presented itself. Then, depending on how serious such a problem became, the individual (or group) faced a decision that was either an ethical issue or a legal matter--or both. The society itself determined ultimately what such an "infraction of the rules" was to be called.

Further, as societies evolved, rapidly or slowly, there was greater or lesser confusion about the subject of ethics. The result seems to have been that--instead of having an impossible ideal confronting the practical necessity of daily life–now a vastly diverse inheritance of ethical ways exists. No matter which ethical way of life one chooses, the others "available" are at least to some degree betrayed. This confusion has been exacerbated because of the complex of ethical systems that the West has inherited (i.e., Hebraic, Christian, Renaissance, Industrial–and now Islam has been added to the mix!).

What might be termed this "philosophic/religious confusion" has historically and inevitably carried over into all aspects of life. Also, it is probably impossible to gain objectivity and true historical perspective on the rapid change that is taking place. Nevertheless, an unprecedented burden of increasing complexity has been imposed on people's understanding of themselves and their world. Many leaders, along with the rest of the population, must certainly be wondering whether the whole affair can be managed.

Down through the 20th century, idealism and realism, followed by pragmatism, were the leading philosophical "stances" in the Western world. However, for some scholars what became known as analytic philosophy emanating from England was gradually superseding the "leading stances" in North America. Let us look at each of these positions in this sequence briefly.

However, sound theory *is* available to humankind through the application of scientific method to problem-solving. So, in such a case, what then is the exact nature of philosophy? Who is really in a position to answer the ultimate questions about the nature of reality? The scientist is, of course. Accordingly, the philosopher must therefore become the servant of science by the employment of conceptual analysis and rational reconstruction of language to help science along. The philosopher has no choice but to be resigned to dealing with important--but lesser!--questions than the origin of the universe, the nature of the human being, and resultant implications for the everyday conduct of this species.

If, therefore, only science and mathematics provide reliable knowledge, philosophy could well then be defined as logical or linguistic analysis. The task of the philosopher accordingly becomes logical or linguistic analysis: the clarification of the meanings of scientific statements. Hence,, interestingly, neither subjectivism nor utilitarianism is the answer either. The former, subjectivism, delved into "feelings of approval," an untenable position to base one's future on. The latter, utilitarianism, also tends to look into the psychological state of happiness or pleasure possibly felt by the acceptance of a recommendation of a specific ethical decision.

As the Western world moves into the 21st Century, the matter of values, ethics, and decision-making is more complex than ever. Graham, in his *Eight theories of ethics* (2004), pointed out that many who seek to enter philosophy's domain are disappointed when they discover that questions about good, evil, and the meaning of life are not answered. Since philosophy's current direction is not so inclined, seeking to ameliorate this dilemma, Graham suggested eight theories of, or approaches to, ethics that he views as having stood the test of time. They are (1) egoism, (2) hedonism, (3) naturalism & virtue theory, (4) existentialism, (5) Kantianism. (6) utilitarianism, (7) contractualism, and (8) religion.

## How Humans Choose Values

Hunter Lewis gave ~~ ·· · ·  · · · · · I · ·¹ I had had earlier back when I was trying to respond to that "dear lady's" request to state "the human values in recreation.". In his outstanding treatment of the subject of human values (1990), Lewis stated that there are six ways that people choose the values they hold:

1. Authority (or "I have faith in the authority of...")

2. Deductive Logic ("Since A is true, B must be true. because B follows from A")

3. Sense Experience ("I know it's true because I saw it, I heard it, I tasted it, I smelled it, or I touched it myself.")

4. Emotion ("I feel that this is true.")

5. Intuition ("After struggling with this problem all day, I went to bed confused and exhausted. The next morning, as I awakened, the solution came to me in a flash–and I just knew it was true.")

6. "Science" ("I tested the hypothesis experimentally and found that it was true."

This listing does seem to "cover the waterfront" insofar as individual decision-making is concerned, but then I realized that when to apply which approach is another matter In addition, I believe there are actually three categories into which these values may be divided: First, those which are personal in the sense that they relates to our immediate relations with family and friends--and our everyday life in society functioning under this or that social or political system. Secondly, as we become professionals in some field of endeavor, we should also explicitly determine our professional value orientation as a fundamental aspect of our relationship to the clients that we serve. Then, thirdly, because of the way the world seems to be going, we are faced with the determination of our social or environmental values. The world is becoming ever-more precarious--and "it's getting real scary out there!"

All of this is not a simple matter to resolve. People are often confused and uncertain in this regard, but frequently they may not recognize or accept the fact that they are confused.  Seemingly they simply have not worked out a coherent, consistent, and reasonably logical approach to the values that they hold–pf think they hold–in life. Most people simply can't express what it was they are working toward in their lives. Typically their values that they held had been achieved *implicitly* and accidentally along the way. Usually they have simply been "handed" down as someone's or some organization's position, creed, or purpose. Only in rare instances has an opportunity been provided for them to think this subject through carefully and systematically so an *explicitly* determined set of values was present for them to bring to bear in decision-making.

Earlier I strove to get to the heart of this massive problem in different ways. I argued that, for several reasons, the child and adolescent in society today are missing out almost completely on a sound "experiential" introduction to ethics. I believe this has created what I call an "ethical decision-making dilemma."

Initially, we need to reconsider *our* values and then re-state **IN SOME TYPE OF GRADUATED OR HIERARCHICAL ORDER** –i.e., exactly what we believe they are in light of the changing times, and then, finally, we will then need to assess more carefully--on a regular basis--whether we are living up to those values we have chosen and so often glibly espouse.

This is true whether we are referring to what takes place in the home, the school system, the church**, OR OUT IN THE EVERYDAY WORLD.** The truth is that typically no systematic instruction in this most important subject is offered at any time. (And I refuse to accept the often-heard "osmosis stance"--that such knowledge is "better caught than taught.") It helps to have people around you who are setting good examples. However, *in the final analysis it is the individual who makes judgments and decisions based on experiences undergone.*

The term ethics is used in three ways: (1) To classify a "way" or pattern of life (e.g., Muslim ethics; (2) As a listing of rules of conduct that is often called a moral code (e.g., professional ethics); and 3) As a description of an investigation or inquiry about rules of conduct or a way of life (e.g., a subdivision of ethics termed meta-ethics = inquiry that treats the meaning and interrelationship of words viewed as moral and ethical.

For example, what is right or wrong; good or bad? Once again, we encounter the question of whether values are objective or subjective (i.e., do values exist whether a person is present to realize them or not? Or, for example, is it people who ascribe value to this or that relationship with others or with their physical environment?

We might ask: "Why is it so important that people give consideration to the topic of values in their lives?" The answer is that values are the major social forces that help to determine the direction a culture will take at any given moment. Choices made are necessarily based on the values and norms of the culture in which people live. Such values titled social values, educational values, scientific values, artistic values, etc. make up the highest level of the social system in a culture. These values represent the "ideal general character" (e.g., social-structured facilitation of individual achievement, equality of opportunity). Remember that overall culture in itself also serves a "pattern-maintenance function" as a society confronts the ongoing functional problems it faces.

Further, the values people hold have a direct relationship to how the nature of the human being is conceived. A number of attempts have been made to define human nature on a rough historical time scale. For example, the human has been conceived in five different ways in historical progression as (1) a rational animal, (2) a spiritual being, (3) a receptacle of knowledge, (4) a mind that can be trained by exercise, and (5) a problem-solving organism (Morris, 1956). Likewise, Berelson and Steiner (1964) traced six behavioral-science images of man and woman throughout recorded history. Identified chronologically these images are: (1) a philosophical image, (2) a Christian image, (3) a political image, (4) an economic image, (5) a psychoanalytic image, and (6) a behavioral-science image.

The "persistent problem" of values has brought confusion. As explained previously rapid change in society had caused general confusion about the subject of ethics. Instead of having an impossible ideal confronting the practical necessity of daily life, we have such a diverse inheritance of ethical ways that no matter which one we choose, the others are at least to some degree betrayed. Obviously, this confusion has been exacerbated because of the complex of moral systems that we have inherited (e.g., Hebraic, Christian, Renaissance, Industrial--and now Islam too, for example).

This philosophic/religious confusion has historically carried over into all aspects of life. Today, it may well be impossible to gain objectivity and true historical perspective on the rapid change that is taking place. Nevertheless, a seemingly unprecedented burden of increasing complexity has been imposed on people's understanding of themselves and their world. Many leaders, along with the rest of us, must certainly be wondering whether the whole affair can be managed.

Further, as we now comprehend that the 20th century was indeed one of marked transition from one era to another, some scholars are beginning to understand that America's quite blind philosophy of optimism about history's malleability and compatibility in keeping with American ideals may turn out to be very shortsighted. At least the weapons stalemate between the U.S.A. and the former U.S.S.R. brought to prominence the importance of nonmilitary determinants (e.g., politics and ideologies). This fact has--and also has **NOT**--sunk into the world's mentality. Most importantly, the world is now witnessing the gradual, but seemingly inevitable, development of a vast ecological crisis that threatens the very existence of the planet known as Earth.

Keeping the above six ways recommended by Lewis firmly in mind, in my teaching of ethical decision making, I finally adopted a three-step or "trivium" approach used by Prof. Richard Fox at Cleveland State University for 30 years as an initial approach to get his students started.

Proceeding on the assumption that a professional person should be able to work out rationally what right and wrong ethical behavior is, he recommended an approach in which there is a progression from the thought of Kant, to Mill, and then to Aristotle. This mat be called a "three-step approach" (or a "trivium") and consists of the application of three "tests" (phrased as questions) to be applied when one wishes to analyze an ethical problem or dilemma. These tests are called: (1) The test of consistency, or universalizability; (2) The test of consequences; and (3) The test of intentions.

A twenty-first century person has a choice to make. He or she must think deeply about the philosophic/religious position he or she holds has validity in the world of the 21st century. If this person's position is the adoption of one of the world's great religions, it would seem vital that he or she should really follow through with the dictates of their particular faith. It would seem to be crucial, however, that the leaders of the various world religions must work for consensus wherever possible on the great issues confronting humankind. Otherwise the perennial confrontations will only lead to frustration and eventual disaster.

## The Function of Values in Society

Careful definition of a particular society is a highly complex task, each one having certain unique qualities while undoubtedly possessing many similarities with other societies. The components of societies are usually described as subsystems (e.g., the economy, the government). In a very real sense these subsystems have been developed to "divide up the work." Before considering a more general discussion of the external environment from the standpoint of resources, the various social organizations, the power structure, and the value structure, there will be a relatively brief presentation of Parsonsian "Action Theory." As described by

Johnson (1969; 1994) as being "a type of empirical system," this particular (grand) theory has a long tradition in the field of sociology. It actually applies to an extremely wide range of systems from relationships between two people to that of total societies.

Initially, to understand this social theory, a person should appreciate that the general action system (implying instrumental activism) is viewed as being composed of four subsystems: (a) cultural system, (b) social system, (c) psychological system, and (d) behavioral-organic system. What this means, viewed from a different perspective, is that explicit human behavior is comprised of aspects that are cultural, social, psychological, and organic. These four subsystems together compose a cybernetic hierarchy of control and conditioning that operates in both directions (i.e., both up and down). (Johnson [1994] explained that an example of a cybernetic system might be a thermostat and an air-conditioning unit [p. 57] . . . . there is an "instrumental activism" occasioned by the "value pattern" of modern societies in which a person's self esteem depends on the extent a contribution is made in some way to life's advancement.)

The first of the subsystems is "culture," which according to Johnson (1969) "provides the figure in the carpet-the structure and, in a sense, the 'programming' for the action system as a whole" (p. 46). The structure of this type of system is typically geared to the functional problems of that level that arise--and so on down the scale, respectively. Thus it is the subsystem of culture that legitimates and also influences the level below it (the social system). Typically, there is a definite strain toward consistency. However, the influence works both upward and downward within the action system, thereby creating a hierarchy of influence or conditioning.

Social life being what it has been and is, it is almost inevitable that strain will develop within the system. Johnson explains this as "dissatisfaction with the level of effectiveness on the functioning of the system in which the strain is felt" (p. 47). Such dissatisfaction may, for example, have to do with particular aspects of a social system as follows: (1) the level of effectiveness of resource procurement; (2) the success of goal attainment; (3) the justice or appropriateness of allocation of rewards or facilities; or (4) the degree to which units of the system are committed to realizing (or maintaining) the values of the system.

Strain may arise at the personality or psychological system level, and the resultant pressure could actually change the structure of the system above (the social system). This is not inevitable, however, because such strain might well be resolved satisfactorily at its own level (so to speak). Usually the pattern consistency of the action system displays reasonable flexibility, and this is especially true at the lower levels. For example, strain might be expressed by deviant behavior or in other ways such as by reduced identification with the social system by the person or group concerned.

Hence, it is *the hierarchy of control and conditioning* that comes into play when the sources of change (e.g., new religious or scientific ideas) begin to cause strain in the larger social systems, whereas the smaller social systems tend to be "strained" by the change that often develops at the personality or psychological system levels. In addition, it is quite apparent that social systems are often influenced considerably by contact with other social systems.

Just as there were four subsystems within the total action system defined by Parsons and others, there are evidently four levels within the subsystem that has been identified as the social system or structure. These levels, proceeding from "highest" to "lowest," are (1) values, (2) norms, (3) the structure of collectivities, and (4) the structure of roles. Typically the higher levels are more general than the lower ones, with the latter group giving quite specific guidance to those segments or units of the particular system to which they apply. These "units" or "segments" are either collectivities or individuals in their capacity as role occupants.

*Values* represent the highest echelon of the social system level of the entire general action system. These values may be categorized into such "entities" as artistic values, educational values, social values, sport values, etc. Of course, all types or categories of values must be values of personalities. The social values of a particular social system are those values that are conceived of as representative of the ideal general character that is desired by those who ultimately hold the power in the system being described. The most important social values in North America, for example, have been (1) the rule of law, (2) the socio-structural facilitation of individual achievement, and (3) the equality of opportunity (Johnson, 1969, p. 48).

*Norms* are the shared, sanctioned rules which govern the second level of the social structure. The average person finds it difficult to separate in his or her mind the concepts of values and norms. Keeping in mind the examples of values offered immediately above, some examples of norms are (1) the institution of private property, (2) private enterprise, (3) the monogamous, conjugal family, and (4) the separation of church and state.

*Collectivities* are interaction systems that may be distinguished by their goals, their composition, and their size. A collectivity is characterized by conforming acts and by deviant acts, which are both classes of members' action that relates to the structure of the system. Interestingly (and oddly) enough, each collectivity has a structure that consists of four levels also (not discussed here). In a pluralistic society one finds an extremely large variety of collectivities that are held together to a varying extent by an overlapping membership constituency. Thus, members of one collectivity can and do exert greater or lesser amounts of influence upon the members of the other collectivities to which they belong.

*Roles* refer to the behavioral organisms (the actual humans) who interact within each collectivity. Each role has a current normative structure specific to it, even though such a role may be gradually changing. (For example, the role of the sport manager or physical activity educator/coach or recreation director could be in a transitory state in that certain second-level norms could be changing, and yet each specific sport manager (or physical educator/coach or recreation director) still has definite normative obligations that are possible to delineate more specifically than the more generalized second-level norms, examples of which were offered above.)

*A hierarchy of control and conditioning.* Finally, these four levels of social structure themselves also compose *a hierarchy of control and conditioning*. As Johnson (p. 49) explains, the higher levels "legitimate, guide, and control" the lower levels, and pressure of both a direct and indirect nature can be--and generally is--employed when the infraction or violation occurs and is known.

A society is the most nearly self-subsistent type of social system and, interestingly enough again, societies or "live systems or personalities" typically have four basic types of functional problems (each with its appropriate value principle) as follows:

1. A pattern-maintenance problem (**L**) that has to do with the inculcation of the value system and the maintenance of the social system's commitment to it,
2. An integration problem (**I**) that is at work to implement the value of solidarity expressed through norms that accordingly regulate the great variety of processes,
3. A goal-attainment problem (**G**) that implements the value of effectiveness of group or collective action on behalf of the social system toward this aim, and
4. An adaptation problem (**A**) whereby the economy implements the value of utility (i.e., the investment-capitalization unit).

The economy of a society is its adaptive subsystem, while the society's form of government (polity) has become known as its goal-attainment subsystem. The integrative and pattern-maintenance subsystems, which do not have names that can be used in everyday speech easily, consist actually of a set or series of processes by which a society's production factors are related, combined, and transformed with utility-the value principle of the adaptive system-as the interim product. These products "packaged" as various forms of "utility" are employed in and by other functional subsystems of the society.

Thus, each subsystem exchanges factors and products, becomes involved as pairs, and engages in what has been called a "double interchange." It is theorized that each subsystem contributes one factor and one product (i.e., one category or aggregate of factors and one category or aggregate of products) to each of the other three functional subsystems. Considered from the standpoint of all the pairs possible to be involved in the interchange, there are therefore six double-interchange systems. Factors and products are both involved in the transformational processes, each being functional for the larger social system. Factors are general and therefore more remote, while products are specific and therefore more directly functional. The performance of the functional requirements has been described as a "circular flow of interchanges," with the factors and products being continuously used up and continuously replaced.

An example of interchange process taking place begins to help us see how this complex circular flow of interchanges occurs. Johnson explains how one of the six interchange systems functions typically to create the political support system in a society. This is how the functional problem of goal-attainment is resolved through the operation of the society's form of government (polity)--that is, the interchange between the polity and the integrative subsystems. "The political process is the set of structured activities that results in the choice of goals and the mobilization of societal resources for the attainment of these goals" (p. 51). First, the integrative system contributes to political accomplishment by achieving a certain degree of consensus and "solidarity." These qualities are "registered" and "delivered" in the form of votes and interest demands. These are, in fact, forms of political support-that is, support from the integrative system to the polity. Conversely, in return, the government (polity) bolsters (integrative) solidarity through political leadership that, in turn, produces binding decisions. Thus, this leadership and the binding decisions can also be considered as "political support"--support from the polity or government to the integrative system (one of the two systems that "produces utility"--i.e., implements one of the four values of which utility is one.)

189

The social significance of interchange analysis is tremendous. The interchange of factors and products identifies the types of processes that somehow must take place in any social system. This scheme specifies also their functional significance and also indicates relations between these processes that are broad but yet important. As was stated earlier, the functional subsystems compose a hierarchy of control and conditioning. Thus, the processes involved are influenced, conditioned, and controlled. These same interchange processes must be going on in any functioning social system, but it should be understood that their specific forms vary greatly. The four levels of a particular social system (i.e., values, norms, collectivities, roles) provide the forms and channels by which any unique social system carries on its functionally necessary processes. Fundamental social change means that some basic transformation has taken, or is taking, place in one or more levels of the social system (structure). Obviously, basic change must inevitably affect the operation of the system in some distinct, measurable way.

Parsons' general action system is then actually an "equilibrium model," but this does not mean that it is necessarily conservative and/or static. As explained above, social systems may, or may not, be in a state of equilibrium, and change is certainly most possible within this theory's framework. This theory is a reasonable, theoretical explanation of how social change can and does take place. Social systems are conceived of as having a normative structure, which may or may not be stable. To understand how to achieve equilibrium within a social system, it is at least theoretically necessary to learn to distinguish between processes that will maintain or change a given social structure. Finally, it is important to understand that sometimes the higher levels of social structure may be maintained (if this is desired and desirable) by understanding how to change one or more of its lower levels. Quite obviously, this last point is most important to anyone serving in a managerial capacity in any organization within a given social system.

## The Value Attached to Physical Activity in World History

The human is born; the human lives; the human moves. To what extent this takes place depends on innumerable occurrences or happenings in a person's life. In Chapters 5 and 6 above, I sought to describe briefly what happened with "human movement in developmental physical activity in exercise, sport, and expressive movement through world history" era by era throughout the past 10,000 years or so. In this summarizing chapter, it seemed best merely to relate *most briefly* what may have happened "stage by stage" in this regard.

*Primitive Society.* Activities of everyday life involving human movement either evolved instinctively or were taught to the young as a means for survival. Dancing and games were probably a part of primitive life to provide recreation and preserve strong healthy bodies. There would typically be a social element involved with such physical activity.

*Early Societies.* Physical activity education was taught by elders to the extent that the young person could carry out normal daily activities. Men prepared physically for militaristic reasons and perhaps to perform in some sporting games, but in the latter to a limited extent. Women's physical activity probably came from daily "living demands." Religious rituals demanded that certain physical activities be performed such as dancing.

*Greece.* Physical (activity) education was highly regarded in ancient Greece and held a prominent place in Greek culture. The development of a healthy body as well as intellectual growth were both part of the Grecian ideal. For the Athenians a balance and (accompanying) harmony between "mind and body" was a most important goal in life. Physical training for the army took precedence in Sparta and was an integral part of a young Spartan's education.. The games arid festivals in Greek life gave young athletes opportunities to compete arid exhibit their physical skills.

*Rome. Regular* physical activity education in the Roman period was encouraged as one way to reach the Roman ideal to become an upstanding citizen willing to serve his nation. Training for the military was and essential part of a child's upbringing to prepare for military service. In Rome's "later period," physical activity education played a minor role in Roman education because it was seen as a degenerate.

*Early Middle Ages.* After the fall of the Roman Empire, Christianity spread rapidly in the West and became a predominant force for the next thousand years. Christianity sought moral, religious and intellectual pursuits more so than it did the physical. As a result, the ascetic way of life prevailed in theory, and the body was denounced because of its "sinful urges." A revival of general education and, to a degree, of physical training occurred during what has been called the Age of Chivalry. Knights were prepared to endure physical and subsequent militaristic stress as well as pay homage to their lord, the Church, and women

*Later Middle Ages.* The Church's overpowering role in society was still felt greatly during the later Middle Ages. As a result, there was little room for formal physical activity education. There were, however, some unorganized sports and games played within the confines of cathedrals and universities. With the rise of humanism, individual concerns were emphasized and proper care and development of the body became more important. Sport and games were used to prepare a boy for war as well as provide some a recreational outlet.

*Early Modern Period.* After the humanistic movement gained widespread recognition over Europe, a shift in educational aims led to a decline of physical education in the early Modern Period. The Reformation did little to revive physical activity within education, but a minority of educators maintained physical training in their curriculum. In education during the Early Modern Period, the study of classical languages and ancient civilizations were increasingly emphasized.

*Age of Enlightenment.* Abrupt changes occurred socially, politically, and in education during the Age of Enlightenment. Naturalism was once again revived which meant that physical activity education was to grow in importance. The Church and state drifted further apart in the control of education. Many new educational theorists were contributing in an effort to develop a more sound philosophy of education. As education became relatively stable in theory, new ideas for physical activity education were included.

*Industrial Age.* During the nineteenth century, physical education emerged more or less as a unique product of the heritage and culture within each nation. For example, in Germany, Friedrich Jahn started the Turnverein movement which emphasized physical training as part of a youth's education. Values within physical education grew in a parallel relationship with social, political, and economic changes. This trend was mostly directed as an outcome of nationalistic feelings.

*20th Century.* In the 20th century governments tried more or less to ensure that all those who receive an education are also given some physical activity education. The field itself within formal education had the following goal: is "The field of physical education (including sport) and the allied fields of health education and recreation should strive to fulfill a significant role in the general educational pattern of the arts, social sciences and natural sciences."(Zeigler, 1977:63) However, the philosophic stances in regard to the importance of physical activity education vary from "essentialistic to progressivistic" depending on a variety of social factors.

## The Kaleidoscopic Value Orientation
## Of Physical Activity Education
## (including Sport)

The historical summary completed above traced physical activity (including sport) very sketchily through history. However, in the subsequent chapter (Chapter 8). I included some *specific* examples depicting the developing kaleidoscopic value orientation of the problems and concerns related to human physical activity in exercise, sport, dance, and physical recreation at all levels and in the public sector. My position is that, individually and collectively, instances such as these serve to "make the case" that the present situation is becoming steadily and increasingly undesirable as we look to the future in the 21st century.

In describing competitive sport in the public sector, it could be classified as amateur, semiprofessional or professional, but somehow the distinction has become ever more "blurred". The category "semiprofessional" is present in practice, but it has never been "officially recognized". Compared to the standards set in their ethical codes for practitioners by the established professions (e.g., education, law, medicine) the only thing that seems to be truly professional about sport in most circumstances is the fact that the participants receive money for their services! In addition, a number of them receive ridiculously high amounts of that legal tender.

In the case of physical (activity) education, however, teachers become members of the education profession, have university degrees, and must be licensed to teach in public education. The problem here is that, despite the mounting of irrefutable evidence as to the benefits of regular exercise and physical recreation through intramural athletics, instruction for "normal" and "special-needs" children and youth in a program mandated in states and provinces varies consistently from good, to fair, to poor, to "non-existent"! The "varsity sport program" for the very few, however, is typically "good" to "excellent."

## Sport as an Anti-value?

To continue, the basic argument I have been making is as follows: *Unless sport participation does "such-and-such" to make people and the society in which they live a better place, such instances must simply be regarded as serving as anti-values!*

What we are finding increasingly is a situation where people seem to be so anxious to escape the *real* world that they are rushing into various sports and similar activities–often involving the possibility of severe personal danger with increasing intensity. They are seemingly often unaware of the potential outcomes of such involvement. (One wonders where the parents are in such instances…)

Coincidently, onrushing science and technology have also become *the tempters of many coaches and athletes.* This possibility has added another dimension to the personal and professional conduct of those people who are unduly anxious for recognition and financial gain.

The premise presented here is, therefore, that beliefs such as these have created a vacuum of positive belief. Hence, sport is overall increasingly becoming more of an anti-value for those who would view *educational **co**mpetitive sport as a life-enhancer* (e.g., those interuniversity sports that are not sustained through gate receipts--golf, tennis, wrestling, swimming, gymnastics, soccer, and almost all of women's sport).

Thus, in an effort to build on Chapter 7 that discussed "what went wrong in the 20th century", Chapter 8 included a kaleidoscope of items that supplement and enhance the claims made in Part 7.

## Physical Education As "All Things to All People" or "Not Too Much To Anyone"

*Shifting attention to the exercise component and the intramural athletics component of the overall physical activity program (including varsity competitive sport),* the development of what was originally the Association for the Advance of Physical Education (with the word "American" added the next year) has been interesting and successful in a variety of ways depending on the interpretation of the word "success." Physical education has been termed a profession, *but it really is a field within the profession of education.* Unfortunately, somehow the connotation of the name–and it reduction to

"PE"–is such that it was not (could not be) used as the name for a profession outside of the educational establishment in the public sector. It is not suitable...

Subsequently within the Association, however, a number of so-called "allied" professions" emerged (i.e., health education, safety education, recreation and park administration, dance (education), athletics (sport), and exercise therapy). The development of these "professions" was undoubtedly influenced down through the years by social forces or societal influences of greater or lesser intensity.

Hess (1959) helped us to somewhat understand how what happened socially and politically enabled him to delineate the leading objectives of physical education from 1900 to 1960:

Hygiene or Health Objective–1900-1919
Socio-Educational Objective–1920-1929
Socio-Recreational Objective–1930-1939
Physical Fitness & Health Objective–1939-1945
'Total Fitness' and International Understanding–
    1946-1957
Disciplinary Development–1959-???

While all of this socio-political development was occurring, a succession of leaders in the field of physical education were attempting to spell out their visions of the  field's objectives in the literature. The following is a chronological list of these leading scholars/practitioners from 1900 to 1950 (see References and Bibliography below, also).:

Hetherington, Wood and Cassidy, Williams, Hughes, Bowen and Mitchell, Nash, Sharman, Wayman. Esslinger, Staley, McCloy, Clark, Cobb, Lynn, Brownell, Scott, Bucher, Oberteuffer, Metheny, Shepherd, Brightbill, Sapora.

An analysis of their recommendations (Zeigler, 1977) resulted on a listing of what could conceivably be called "common denominators" in program development:

Movement Fundamentals
Regular Exercise
Health & Safety Education
Physical Recreation

Physical Fitness
Competitive Sport
Therapeutic Exercise

Recently I have expanded a bit on this list of so-called "common denominators" for physical activity education in the hope that there might be considerable agreement in the developed world. These proposed common denominators are as follows:

1. That regular physical activity education (including related health information) be *required* for all children and young people up to and including sixteen years of age.
2. That human movement fundamentals through various dance and other expressive activities be included in the elementary, middle, and high school curricula.
3. That progressive standards for physical vigor and endurance for people of all ages be developed from prevailing norms.
4. That the physical activity & health educator's responsibility should be *a full-time one*.

   (Note: The implication here is that any sport coaching involvement on his or her part would be the same as that with any other teacher in the school based on the practices of the community involved.)

5. That remediable bodily defects be corrected where possible through exercise therapy. Referral to the family doctor may be necessary to initiate a remedial program. Where possible, adapted sport and physical recreation experiences should be offered.
6. That boys and girls (and young men and women) have an experience in competitive sport at some stage of their development.
7. That people develop certain positive attitudes toward their own health in particular and toward community hygiene in general. Basic health knowledge should be integral part of the school curriculum.

   (Note: This "common denominator" should be a specific objective of the profession of physical activity education only to the extent that it relates to developmental physical activity.)

8. That sport, dance, exercise, and play can make a most important contribution throughout life toward the worthy use of leisure.

9. That character and/or personality development is vitally important to the development of the young person. Therefore, it is especially important that all human movement experience in sport, dance, exercise, and play at the various educational levels be guided by men and women with high professional standards and ethics.

Despite the above, there is ongoing evidence that "all is not well." In 2006 Eleanor Randolph, in "The Big, Fat American Kid Crisis...and Things We Should Do About It" explained that:

> The problem is all too obvious. At the mall, the movie theater or the airport, the evidence appears in the flesh – altogether too much of it. Americans are now officially supersized, overweight, obese even. This is true of almost two thirds of American adults, but what is more alarming, it is also true of millions of American children. The "little ones" aren't so little any rnore.
>
> Yes, they are gently labeled "chunky," "husky" or "plus-sized" by the clothes marketers who are adding larger and larger sizes to the children's racks. But these euphemisms can't cover up the unpleasant reality that too many of our kids are so dangerously overweight that they are spilling out of their childhood too chubby for their car seats or too uncomfortable as they squeeze into their little desks at elementary school. But the real problem is not aesthetics or the need to save classroom space. Childhood obesity has become a national medical crisis.
>
> Over the last 30 years, obesity rates have doubled among pre-school children and tripled for those aged 6 to 11. For those added pounds, the young are starting to pay a terrible price. Adult diabetes has rapidly become a childhood disease. Pediatricians are seeing high cholesterol and high blood pressure and other grown-up problems in their patients. Teachers and school psychiatrists are coping with a plague of shame and distress among children whose size subjects them to hazing and other cruelties by their classmates.

There is some evidence that more people are becoming aware of the two problems I have been describing. *The Wall Street Journal* (2010 06 09) summarized a report emanating from the National Association for Sport and Physical Education and the American Heart Association stating that there was a slight improvement in the percentage of states requiring physical education since that of a survey carried out in 2006. *However, most of the states have no requirement as to the time allotment of such a requirement—and half of them permits waivers, exemptions, and substitutions…"*

Reports of this type could go on endlessly, but I'll end with a conclusion stated in *Active Living Research*, a national program of the Robert Wood Johnson Foundation (Fall, 2007, Research Brief):

> In schools across the United States, physical education has been substantially reduced—and in some cases completely eliminated—in response to budget concerns and pressures to improve academic test scores. Yet the available evidence shows that children who are physically active and fit tend to perform better in the classroom, and that daily physical education does not adversely affect academic performance. Schools can provide outstanding learning environments while improving children's health through physical education.

The situation in Canada doesn't appear to be much better. Jo-Ann Fellows, a columnist in Fredericton, NB, Canada, recently wrote:

> For the fourth year in a row, a failing grade has been handed out to the whole country. Only 12 per cent of Canadian children and youth are meeting the guideline of 90 minutes per day.

> The report card was issued by Active Healthy Kids Canada. Its mandate states that it provides "… the evidence base for our communications and issue advocacy work to increase support for quality, accessible and enjoyable physical activity participation experiences for young people across Canada."

(See <dailygleaner.canadaeast.com/search/article/1056903>)

Following these brief analyses of (1) the prevailing situation in public-sector sport and (2) physical (activity) education (including athletics) within the education establishment, I have included a number of examples to support the overall position being taken here.

## Future Societal Scenarios

Walter Truett Anderson, president of the American Division of the World Academy of Art and Science, has sketched four different scenarios as postulations for the future of earthlings in this ongoing adventure of civilization. In an essay titled "Futures of the Self," taken from *The Future of the Self: Inventing the Postmodern Person* (1997), Anderson argued convincingly that current trends are adding up to a future identity crisis for humankind. The creation of the present "modern self," he explains, began with Plato, Aristotle, and with the rights of humans in Roman legal codes.

The developing conception of self bogged down in the Middle Ages, but fortunately was resurrected in the Renaissance Period described by many historians as the second half of The Middle Ages. Since then the human "self" has been advancing like a "house afire" as the Western world has gone through an almost unbelievable transformation. As it happened, scientists like Galileo and Copernicus influenced philosophers such as Descartes and Locke to foresee a world in which the self was invested with human rights.

*"One World, Many Universes."* Anderson's "One World, Many Universes" version is the most likely to occur. This is a scenario characterized by high economic growth, steadily increasing technological progress, and globalization combined with high psychological development. Such psychological maturity, he predicts, will be possible for a certain segment of the world's population because "active life spans will be gradually lengthened through various advances in health maintenance and medicine" (pp. 251-253)

Nevertheless, a problem has developed with this dream of individual achievement of inalienable rights and privileges, one that looms large in the early years of this new century. The modern self that was envisioned by Descartes, a rational, integrated self that Anderson likens to Captain Kirk at the command post of Starship Enterprise, appears to be having an identity crisis. The image of this bold leader (he or she!) taking us fearlessly into the great unknown has begun to fade as alternate scenarios for the future of life on Earth are envisioned. In a world where globalization and economic "progress" seemingly must be rejected because of catastrophic environmental concerns or "demands," the bold-future image could well "be replaced by a post-modern self; de–centered, multidimensional, and changeable" (p. 50).

Captain Kirk–as he "boldly went where no man had gone before"--this time to rid the world of terrorists and evil leaders), now faces a second crucial change. As leaders seek to shape the world of the 21st century, based on Anderson's analysis, there is another force–the systemic-change force mentioned above–that is shaping the future. This all-powerful force may well exceed the Earth's ability to cope. As gratifying as such factors as "globalization along with economic growth" and "psychological development" may seem to the folks in a coming "One-World, Many Universes" scenario, there is a flip side to this prognosis. Anderson identifies this image as "The Dysfunctional Family" scenario. All of these benefits of so-called progress are highly expensive and available now only to relatively few of the six billion plus people on earth. Anderson foresees this affairs splintering into (1) "a world of modern people happily doing their thing; of modern people still obsessed with progress, economic gain, and organizational bigness; and (2) of postmodern people being trampled and getting angry" (p. 51). As people get angrier, Anderson envisions present-day terrorism in North America seeming like child's play.

## The Field Has Reached a Crucial Stage

There is good evidence that the next ten to fifteen years will be crucial ones for the field of physical (activity) education and (so-called) educational sport. This is true because the profession is not growing and developing as rapidly and strongly as it should be in a society where the idea of change must now become our watchword. View it as you will, it is impossible to refute the thought that change, like death and taxes, is here to stay.

Diagnosis of the present situation leads to the belief that the "developmental physical activity" professed by the field of physical activity education (including educational/recreational sport--as it has been known and promoted--is structurally deficient in what may be called the field's architecture. Many people recognize that something is wrong, but most of them don't appear to understand the extent of the malady that has gradually infected a still embryonic profession.

The situation appears to be as follows: Throughout the land school programs of physical activity education inculcating theory and practice of developmental activity education at all levels are either good, bad, indifferent, or completing lacking! The fourteen "principles of physical activity education" that I have outlined provide indisputable evidence that regular physical activity is required for vital life efficiency and longevity, but the field of education and the public that may provide it for youth (or not!) have assumed a sort of "I know it's true approach, but

200

it's costly, a nuisance, and 'sweaty' too–not to mention that it interferes with the professional sport that I am watching on television.".

At the same time, as far as people's children are concerned, there are all sorts of varsity sport teams "for the very few" competing at all levels of education throughout the length and breadth of the land. The world is becoming increasingly "sport-happy" as we hear or read daily that poor health and physical-activity practices are creating a situation where children and youth the coming generation will die before their parents do!

Still further, a recent study in Scotland points out that the situation with adults has reached a "ridiculous stage" as well. It was stated that 97.5% of adults there are "likely to be cigarette smokers, heavy drinkers, physically inactive, overweight or have a poor diet. These findings may be even worse because they were self reported in a 2003 Scottish Health Survey published in *BMC Public Health* *(The Vancouver Sun, 2010, 06, 12, C8).*

## What Should We Do in the 21st Century?

Note: These recommendations to the profession of physical (activity) education originally appeared on pp. 340-346 of the author's 2005 *History and Status of American Physical Education and Educational Sport* (Victoria, BC: Trafford). Based on my various efforts to analyze the events of the final half of the 20th century, these 20 recommendations are offered again for the consideration of the field of physical activity education including educational sport in the 21st century. For any parent who might be reading these words, they may help him or her to comprehend the situation better,

1. *A Sharper Image.* In the past the field of physical (activity) education and educational sport tried to be "all things to all people." Now it should sharpen its image and improve the quality of its efforts by focusing primarily on *developmental physical activity*--specifically, human motor performance in sport, exercise, and related expressive movement. As we sharpen our image, we should make a strong effort to include those who are working in the private agency and commercial sectors as members of the profession. This means that we will extend our efforts to promote the finest type of developmental physical activity for people of all ages whether they be members of what are considered to be "normal, accelerated, or special" populations.

2. *Our Field's Name.* All sorts of name changes have been implemented at the university level (1) to explain either what people think we are doing or should be doing, or (2) to camouflage the presumed "unsavory" connotation of the term "physical education" that evidently conjures up the notion of a "dumb jock" working with the lesser part of a tri-partite human body. We should continue to focus primarily on *developmental physical activity* as defined immediately above while moving toward an acceptable working term for our profession. In so doing, we should keep in mind the field's or subject-matter's bifurcated nature in that it has both theoretical and practical (or disciplinary and professional) aspects. At the moment the terms "kinesiology" and "physical education" are in vogue. A desirable name for the profession might be *physical activity education* with the term *developmental physical activity* as the field of study or discipline. We could delineate this further by including exercise, sport, and expressive movement as aspects of the field.

3. *A Tenable Body of Knowledge.* Various social forces and professional concerns have placed us in a position where we don't know where or what our body of knowledge is. As a profession we will strongly support the idea of disciplinary definition and the continuing development of *a body of knowledge* based on such a consensual definition. From this must come a merging of tenable scientific theory in keeping with societal values. Through computer technology we can now gradually, steadily, and increasingly provide our members with the knowledge as ordered generalizations in an evolving manner to help them perform as top-flight professionals. As qualified professionals, we simply must possess the requisite knowledge, competencies, and skills necessary to provide developmental physical activity services of a high quality to the public.

4. *Our Own Professional Associations.* There is currently insufficient support of *our own* professional and scholarly associations for a variety of reasons. We need to develop voluntary and mandatory mechanisms that relate membership in professional and scholarly organizations both directly and indirectly to stature within the overall field. We simply must now commit ourselves also to work tirelessly and continually to promote the welfare of professional practitioners who are serving the public in areas that we represent. Additionally, it may be necessary to exert any available pressures to encourage people to give first priority to our own groups (as opposed to those of related disciplines and/or allied professions). The logic behind this dictum is that our own survival must come first for us!

5. *Professional Licensing.* Most teachers/coaches in the schools, colleges, and universities are seemingly protected indefinitely by the shelter of the all-embracing

teaching profession. Now, additionally, we should now move rapidly and strongly to seek official recognition of our endeavors in public, semi-public, and private agency work and in commercial organizations relating to developmental physical activity *through professional licensing at the state and provincial level.* Further, we should encourage individuals to apply for voluntary registration as qualified practitioners at the federal level. This should be encouraged no matter with what terminology they classify their efforts (e.g., personal trainer).

6. *Harmony Within The Field.* An unacceptable series of gaps and misunderstandings has developed among those in our field concerned primarily with the bio-scientific aspects of human motor performance, those concerned with the social-science and humanities aspects, those concerned with the general education of all students, and those concerned with the professional preparation of physical activity educators/coaches--all at the community or university level. We will now strive to work for *a greater balance and improved understanding* among these essential entities within the field/discipline.

7. *Harmony Among The "Allied Professions".* The field of physical education spawned a number of allied professions down through the years of the 20th century. *We should now strive to comprehend what they claim that they do professionally, and where there may be a possible overlap with what we as educators or practicing professionals claim that we do.* Where disagreements prevail, they should be ironed out to the greatest extent possible at the national level.

8. *The Relationship With University Athletics/Sport.* A wedge is being driven increasingly between units of kinesiology/physical education and interuniversity athletics. This is true in those educational institutions where gate receipts are increasingly becoming a stronger factor. Such a rift serves no good purpose and is counter to the best interests of both groups. *We will now work for greater understanding and harmony with those people who are primarily interested in the promotion of highly organized athletics. At the same time it is imperative that we do all in our power to maintain athletics in a sound educational perspective within our schools, colleges, and universities.*

9. *The Relationship with Intramurals and Recreational Sport.* Intramurals and recreational sport is in a transitional state at present in that it has proved that it is "here to stay" at the college and university level. Nevertheless, intramurals hasn't really taken hold yet, generally speaking, at the high-school or middle-school levels, despite the fact that it has a great deal to offer the large majority of students in what may truly be called *recreational* or even *educational* sport. There is a minority of administrators functioning at the college level who would like to adopt the term

"campus recreation" as their official designation. However, this is not an appropriate designation unless this program encompasses all recreational activities on campus. it appears to be impractical and inadvisable to attempt to subsume *all* non-curricular activities on campus under one division or unit. Further, the various departments and divisions of ought to work for consensus on the idea that *intramurals and recreational sport is co-curricular in nature* and deserve regular funding as laboratory experience in the same manner that general education course experiences in physical education receive their funding for instructional purposes.

10. *Guaranteeing Equal Opportunity.* Because "life, liberty, and the pursuit of happiness" are guaranteed to all, as a profession we should move positively and strongly to see to it that *equal opportunity* is indeed provided to the greatest possible extent to women, to minority groups, and to special populations as they seek to improve the quality of their lives through the finest type of experience in the many activities of our field.

11. *The Kinesiology/Physical Education Identity.* In addition to the development of the so-called allied professions (e.g., health education in the second quarter of the twentieth century), we witnessed the advent of a disciplinary thrust in the 1960s that was followed by a splintering of many of the various "knowledge components" and subsequent formation of many different scholarly societies. These developments have undoubtedly weakened the core field of physical (activity) education as it is now called within schools. It appears that the term "kinesiology," along with improved scholarly effort, has strengthened the field's status at the university level. Thus, it is now more important than ever that we *hold high the developmental physical education identity.* Additionally we should re-affirm and delineate even more carefully our relationship with our "allied professions".

12. *Applying a Competency Approach.* Considering the failures and inconsistencies of longstanding educational teaching methodology, *we will as a field explore diligently the educational possibilities of a competency approach* as it might apply to general education, to professional preparation, and to all aspects of our professional endeavor in public, semi-public, private, and commercial agency endeavors. This means that all education is experiential in the sense that laboratory experiences characterize all course instruction.

13. *Managing the Enterprise.* All professionals in our unique field of developmental are managers--but to varying degrees. The "one course in administration" approach with no laboratory or internship experience of earlier times is simply not sufficient now or for the future with those positions that are

"substantively" administrative in nature.. There is an urgent need to apply a competency approach in the preparation (as well as in the continuing education) of those who will serve as managers either within educational circles or elsewhere in the society at large.

14. *Ethics and Morality in Physical Activity Education (including Educational Sport.* In the course of the development of the best professions, the various, embryonic professional groups have gradually become conscious of the need for a set of professional ethics--that is, a set of professional *obligations* that are established as *norms* for practitioners in good standing to follow. Our unique field needs both a creed and a detailed code of ethics right now as we move ahead in our development. Such a move is important because, generally speaking, ethical confusion prevails in North American society. Development of a sound code of ethics, combined with steady improvement in the three essentials of a fine profession (i.e., [a] an extensive period of training, [b] a significant intellectual component that must be mastered before the profession is practiced, and [c] a recognition by society that the trained person can provide a basic, important service to its citizens) would relatively soon place us in a much firmer position to claim that we are indeed members of a fine discipline and accompanying professional field.)

15. *Reunifying the Profession's Integral Elements.* Because there now appears to be reasonable agreement that our field, one that is now called by such a multitude of often incongruent names, is concerned primarily with developmental physical activity as manifested in human motor performance in sport, exercise, and related expressive movement, *we will now work for the reunification of those elements of our profession that should be uniquely ours within our disciplinary definition.*

16. *Cross-Cultural Comparison and International Understanding.* We have done reasonably well in the area of international relations within the Western world due to the solid efforts of many dedicated people over a considerable period of time. However, we need now to redouble our efforts to make cross- cultural comparisons of kinesiology and physical education while reaching out for international understanding and cooperation. Much greater understanding on the part of all of the concepts of 'communication,' 'diversity,' and 'cooperation' is required for the creation of a better life for all in a *peaceful* world. Our field, both its disciplinary and professional aspects, can contribute significantly toward this long range objective.

17 *Permanency and Change.* The "principal principles" espoused for physical education and sport in the 1950s by the late Dr. Arthur Steinhaus of George

Williams College still apply basically to our professional endeavors (i.e., the overload principle, the principle of reversibility, the principle of integration and integrity, and the principle of the priority of man and woman). *We will continue to emphasize that which is timeless in our work, while at the same time accept the inevitability of certain societal change.*

18. *Improving the Quality of Life.* Our field is unique within education and in society. Since fine living and professional success involve so much more than the important verbal and mathematical skills, we will emphasize strongly that education is a lifelong enterprise. Further, we will stress that *the quality of life can be improved significantly through the achievement of a higher degree of kinetic awareness and through regular, heightened experiences in sport, exercise, and related expressive movement.*

19. *ImprovingtheLengthofLife.* Mounting evidence indicates that people will also live longer if they live life actively and make wise exercise choices. Despite this increased longevity, healthcare costs will be reduced because of the ongoing health benefits derived from such regular involvement. So, in addition to promoting the idea that "quality of life" will be heightened, we will stress also *the practical idea that lowered healthcare costs will accompany this increased length-of-life "bonus" that regular physical activity provides.*

20. *Reasserting Our "Will to Win".* The developments of the past 50 years have undoubtedly created a state of unease within the discipline and the profession. They have also raised doubts on the part of some as to our possession of a "will to win" through the achievement of the highest type of professional status *We pledge ourselves anew to make still greater efforts to become vibrant and stirring through absolute dedication and commitment in our disciplinary and professional endeavors.* Ours is a high calling as we seek to improve the quality of life for all through the finest type of human motor performance in sport, exercise, and related expressive movement.

## Concluding Statement

Those who read these words and who are truly concerned about the future of humankind, wherever you may be, are strongly urged to get involved now with the reforms that seem so necessary

In the immediate future, please seek the answer to two fundamental questions. The response to the first question might well cause action to be taken in the future to answer question #2. These questions are:

(1) in what ways can we institute related physical activity accurately to learn if sport is--**or is not**--fulfilling its presumed role and providing value as a presumably beneficent social institution?

(2)--depending on whether the answer to #1 is positive or negative, will you then also have the motivation to do your utmost to help related physical activity education (and related health education) achieve what should be its rightful place in society?

The author's stance is obviously that:

*Human physical activity, broadly interpreted and experienced under wise educational or recreational conditions, can indeed provide value and be a worthwhile social institution contributing vitally to the well being, ongoing health and longevity of humankind?*

## References and Bibliography

Aburdene, P. & Naisbitt, J. (1992). *Megatrends for women.* NY: Villard Books. 388 p.

Adams, G.B. (1922) *Civilization during the Middle Ages.* NY: Charles Scribner's Sons.

Amara, R. (1981). The futures field. The Futurist, February.

American Alliance for Health, Physical Education, and Recreation (Spring 1957) Statement of policies and procedures for girls' and women's sport. *JOHPER*, 28, 6:57-58.

American Alliance for Health, Physical Education, Recreation and Dance (1962) *Professional preparation in health education, physical education, recreation education. Report of national conference.* Washington, DC: Author.

American Alliance for Health, Physical Education, Recreation and Dance. (1974). *Professional preparation in dance, physical education, recreation education, safety education, and school health education.* Report on national conference. Washington, DC: Author.

Anderson, W.T. (1996). *The Fontana postmodernism reader,* London: Fontana Press.

Anderson, W.T. (1997). *The future of the self: Inventing the postmodern person.* NY: Tarcher/Putnam.

Artz, F.B. (1981). *The mind of the Middle Ages.* (3rd Ed.). Chicago: Univ. of Chicago Press.

Asimov, I. (1970). The fourth revolution. *Saturday Review.* Oct. 24, 17-20.

Ayer, A. J. (1984) *Philosophy in the twentieth century.* NY: Vintahe.


Bagley, J.J. (1961). *Life in medieval England.* London: B.T. Batsford.

Ballou, R.B. (1965). *An analysis of the writings of selected church fathers to A.D. 394 to reveal attitudes regarding physical activity.* Doctoral dissertation, University of Oregon.

Barber, R. (1975). *The knight and chivalry.* Totowa, NJ: Rowman and Littlefield.

Barker, J. (1986). *The tournament in England, 1100-1400.* Suffolk: Boydell and Brewer.

Barney, R.K. (1985). The hailed, the haloed, and the hallowed: Sport heroes and their qualities--An analysis and hypothetical model for their commemoration. In

Sport History Official Report, Olympic Scientific Congress (N. Mueller & J. Ruehl, eds.). Niederhausen, FRG: Schors-Verlag.

Barrett, W. (1959). *Irrational man: A study in existential philosophy*. Garden City, NY: Doubleday.

Barrows, I.C., ed. (1899) *Proceedings of the Conference on Physical Training*. Boston: Press of G. H. Ellis.

Barzun, J. (1974). *The use and abuse of art*. Princeton: Princeton Univ. Press.

Bazzano, C. (1973). *The contribution of the Italian Renaissance to physical education*. Doctoral dissertation, Boston University.

Beeler, J. (1966). *Warfare in England*. Ithaca, NY: Cornell University Press.

Bennett, B.L. (1962). Religion and physical education. Paper presented at the Cincinnati Convention of the AAHPER, April 10.

Bentley, E. (1969). *The cult of the superman*. MA: Gloucester.

Bereday, G.Z.F. (1964). *Comparative method in education* (see pp. 11-27). New York: Holt, Rinehart and Winston.

Bereday, G.Z.F. (1969). Reflections on comparative methodology in education, 1964-1966. In M.A. Eckstein & H.J. Noah (Eds.), *Scientific investigations in comparative education* (pp. 3-24). New York: Macmillan.

Berelson, B. and Steiner, G. A. (1964). *Human Behavior*. NY: Harcourt, Brace, Jovanovich.

Berman, M. (2001) *The twilight of American culture*. NY: W.W. Norton.

Blinde, E.M. & McCallister, S.G. (1999). Women, disability, and sport and physical fitness activity: The intersection of gender and disability dynamics. *Research Quarterly for Sport and Exercise*, 70, 3, 303-312.

Bookwalter, K.W., & Bookwalter, C.W. (1980). *A review of thirty years of selected research on undergraduate professional preparation physical education programs in the United States*. Unionville, IN: Author.

Boorstin, D.J. (1961). *The image: Or what happened to the American dream*. London: Weidenfeld and Nicolson.

Booth, F.W., & Chakravarthy, M.V. (2002). Cost and consequences of sedentary living: New battleground for an old enemy. *Research Digest (PCPFS)*, 3, 16, 1-8.

Borgman, A. (1993) *Crossing the postmodern divide*. Chicago: The University of Chicago Press.

Borradori, G. (1994). *The American philosopher*. Chicago: Univ.of Chicago Press.

Bottomley, F. (1979). *Attitudes toward the body in Western Christendom*. London: Lepus.

Bradbury, J. (1985). *The medieval archer*. NY: St. Martin's Press.

Brady, M. (March/April 1994). Correspondence. *Utne Reader*, 62: 6-7.

Broekhoff, J. ((1973). Chivalric education in the Middle Ages. In E. F. Zeigler, Ed. & Au.), *A history of sport and physical education to 1900* (pp. 225-234). Champaign, IL: Stipes.

Bronowski, J. & Mazlish, B. (1975). *The Western intellectual tradition: From Leonardo to Hegel*. New York: Harper & Row,

Broudy, H.S. (1961). *Building a philosophy of education*. 2nd ed. Englewood Cliffs, NJ: Prentice-Hall.

Brubacher, J. S. (1966). *A history of the problems of education*. (2nd Ed.). NY: McGraw-Hill.

Brubacher, J. S. (1969). *Modern philosophies of education* (4th ed.). New York: McGraw-Hill.

Bury, J. B. (1955). *The idea of progress*. New York: Dover.

Butler, H. (1975). Lifting the veil of ignorance with a philosophy of commitment. *Philosophy in Context*, 4: 111-117.

Butler, J. D. (1957) *Four philosophies*. (Rev. Ed.). NY: Harper.

Butts, R. F. (1947). *A cultural history of education*. New York: McGraw-Hill.


Calin, W. (1966). *The epic quest*. Baltimore: Johns Hopkins Press.

Carlyle, T. (n.d.). *Heroes, hero worship and the heroic in history*. NY: A. L. Burt.

Carter, J.M. (May 1980). *Sport in the Bayeux Tapestry*, Canadian Journal of Sport History, XI, 1: 36-60.

Carter, J.M. (1981). *Ludi medi aevi: Studies in the history of medieval sport*. Manhattan, KS: Military Affairs Publishing.

Carter, J.M. (1988). *Sports and pastimes of the Middle Ages*. Lanham, MD: University Press of America.

Carter, J.M. (1992).*Medieval games; Sports and recreations in feudal society*. Westport, CT: Greenwood.

Castiglione, B. (1959). *The book of the courtier* (C.S. Singleton, trans.). NY: Doubleday.

Caxton, W. (1926). *The book of the order of chyvalry*. In A.T. Bayles, (Ed.). London: Oxford University Press.

Champion, S.G. & Short, D. (1951). *Readings from the world religions*. Boston: Beacon.

Chaucer, G. (1991). *The Canterbury tales*. (Begun in 1387). NY:

QPBC.

Childs, J.L. (1931). *Education and the philosophy of experimentalism*. NY: Appleton-Century-Crofts.

Clephan, C.R. (1919). *The tournament: Its periods and phases*. NY: Ungar.(Clepham, R.C.??)

*Columbia Encyclopedia, The New* (W.H. Harvey & J.S. Levey, Eds.). (1975). NY: Columbia University Press.

Commager, H.S. (1961). A quarter century--Its advances. *Look*, 25, 10 (June 6), 80-91.

Commission on Tests, College Entrance Examination Board. (Nov. 2, 1970). *The New York Times*.

Conant, J.B. (1963). *The education of American teachers* (pp. 122-123). New York: McGraw-Hill.

Contributions of physical activity to human well-being. (May, 1960) *Research Quarterly*, 31, 2 (Part II):261-375.

Cornish, F.W. (1901). *Chivalry*. NY: Macmillan.

Cosentino, F. & Howell, M.L. (1971). *A history of physical education in Canada*. Don Mills, Ont.: General Publishing Co.

Coulton, G.G. (1960). *Medieval village, manor and monastery*. NY: Harper.

Cowell, C.C. (1960). The contributions of physical activity to social development. *Research Quarterly*, 31, 2 (May, Part II), 286-306.

Cryderman, K. (2001). Sport's culture of adultery. *The Vancouver Sun* (Canada), August 21, C5.

Crossland, J. (1956). *Medieval French literature*. Oxford: Basil Blackwell.

Cuff, J.H. (1983). Just regular guys. *The Globe and Mail* (Toronto), Aug. 20, 3.

Cummins, J. *The hound and the hawk: The art of medieval hunting*. NY: St. Martin's Press.

Czikszentmihalyi, M. (1993). *The evolving self: A psychology for the third millenium*. NY: Harper Perennial.


Davis, E.C. (1961). *The philosophical process in physical education*. Philadelphia: Lea & Febiger. (Includes several excellent analyses by Roger Burke.)

Davis, E.C. (1963). *Philosophies fashion physical education*. Dubuque, IA: Wm.C.Brown.

DeMott, B. (1969). How existential can you get? *The New York Times Magazine*, March 23, pp. 4, 6, 12, 14.

Depauw, K.P. (1997). The (in)visibility of disability: Cultural contexts and "sporting bodies," *Quest*, 49, 416-430.

Dewey, J. (1938). *Logic, the theory of inquiry*. NY: Holt, Rinehart and Winston.

Dubin, R. (1978) <u>Theory building</u>. NY: The Free Press.

Durant, W. (1938). The story of philosophy. (New rev. ed.). NY: Garden City.

Durant, W. (1950). *The age of faith.* NY: Simon and Schuster.

Durant, W. & Durant, A. (1968). *The lessons of history.* New York: Dover.

Ellfeldt, L.E., & Metheny, E. (1958). Movement and meaning: Development of a general theory." *Research Quarterly*, 29, 264-273.

Elliott, R. (1927). *The organization of professional training in physical education in state universities.* New York: Columbia Teachers College.

*Encarta World English Dictionary, The.* (1999). NY: St. Martin's Press.

*Encyclopedia of Philosophy, The* (P. Edwards, Ed.). (1967). (8 vols.). NY: Macmillan & Free Press.

English, E. (1984). Sport, the blessed medicine of the Renaissance. In *Proceedings of the North American Society for the Study of Sport History* (D. Wiggins, Ed.). Kansas State University Press, Manhattan.

Eyler, M.H. (1956). *Origins of some modern sports.* Ph.D. dissertation, University of Illinois, Champaign-Urbana.


Fahlberg, L.L., & Fahlberg L.A. (1994). A human science for the study of movement: An integration of multiple ways of knowing. *Research Quarterly for Exercise and Sport.* 65, 100-109.

Fairs, J. R. (1973). The influence of Plato and Platonism on the development of physical education in Western culture. In E. F. Zeigler (Ed. & Au.), *A history of sport and physical education to 1900,* pp. 155-166 Champaign, IL: Stipes.

Feibleman, J. (1973). *Understanding philosophy.* NY: Dell.

Feschuk, S. (2002). Night of the Olympic dead. *National Post* (Canada), Feb. 16, B10.

Finley, M. I. (1965) The world of Odysseus. NY: Viking.

Fishwick, M. (1969). The hero, American style. NY: David McKay.

Flach, J. (1904). Chivalry. In *Medieval civilization* (D. Munro & G. Sellery, Eds.). NY: Century.

Flath, A.W. (1964). *A history of relations between the National Collegiate Athletic Association and the Amateur Athletic Union of the United States (1905-1963).* Champaign, IL: Stipes.

Forsyth, I.H. (April 1978). The theme of cockfighting in Burgundian

Romanesque sculpture. *Speculum*: 252-282.

Fraleigh, W.P. (1970). Theory and design of philosophic research in physical education. *Proceedings of the National College Physical Education Association for Men,* Portland, OR, Dec. 28.

Fraleigh, W.P. (1984). *Right actions in sport.* Champaign, IL: Human Kinetics.

Froissart, J. (1842). *Chronicles of England, France, Spain, and the adjoining countries.* (2 Vols.). (T. Johnes, trans.). London: Smith.


Gautier, L. (1989). *Chivalry.* London: Bracken. (This book was originally published as La Chevalrie in 1883 in Paris.)

Geiger, G.R. (1955). An experimentalistic approach to education. In N.B. Henry (Ed.), *Modern philosophies and education* (Part I). Chicago: Univ. of Chicago Press.

Gerzon, M. (1982). A choice of heroes. Boston: Houghton Mifflin.

Gies, F. (1964). *The knight in history.* NY: Harper & Row.

Gimpel, J. (1976). *The medieval machine: The industrial revolution of the Middle Ages.* NY; Holt, Rinehart and Winston.

Glasser, W. (1972). *The identity society.* NY: Harper & Row.

Glassford, R.G. (1970) *Application of a theory of games to the transitional Eskimo culture.* Ph.D. dissertation, University of Illinois, Urbana.

Good, C.F., & Scates, D.E. (1954). *Methods of research* New York: Appleton-Century-Crofts.

Goode, W.J. The celebration of heroes. Berkeley, CA: Univ. of California Press.

Green. H. (1986). *Fit for America.* Baltimore: The Johns Hopkins University Press..

Greene, T.M. (1955). A liberal Christian idealist philosophy of education. In N.B. Henry (Ed.), *Modern Philosophies of education.* Chicago, Univ. of Chicago Press.

Guttman, A. (1986). *Sports spectators.* NY: Columbia University Press.


Hahm, C. H., Beller, J .M., & Stoll, S. K. (1989). *The Hahm-Beller Values Choice Inventory.* Moscow, Idaho: Center for Ethics, The University of Idaho.

Handlin, O. et al. (1967). Harvard guide to American history. NY: Atheneum

Hartshorne, C. (1975). The nature of philosophy. *Philosophy in Context* 4: 7-16.

Haskins, C. H. (1995). *The Normans in European history.* NY: Barnes &

Noble.

Hayes, C. (1961). *Nationalism: A religion*. New York: Macmillan.

Heilbroner, R. L. (1960). *The future as history*. New York: Harper & Row.

Heinemann, F. H. (1958). *Existentialism and the modern predicament*. NY: Harper & Row.

Henry, J. (1963). Culture against man. NY: Random House.

Henricks, T. S. (1982). Sport and social hierarchy in medieval England. *Journal of Sport History*, IX, 2: 20-37.

Henricks, T. S. (1991) *Disputed pleasures: Sport and society in pre-industrial England*. Westport, CT: Greenwood.

Henry, N. B., ed. (1942). *The Forty-First Yearbook of the National Society for the Study of Education*. (Part I). Chicago: University of Chicago Press.

Hershkovits, M. J. (1955). *Cultural anthropology*. New York: Knopf.

Hess, F. A. (1959). *American objectives of physical education from 1900 to 1957 assessed in light of certain historical events*. Ph.D. dissertation, New York University.

Hocking, W.E. (1928). *The meaning of God in human experience*. New Haven, CT: Yale University Press.

Hoernle, R. F. A. (1927). *Idealism as a philosophy*. NY: Doubleday.

Holmes, U. T. *Daily living in the twelfth century* Madison, WI: Univ. of Wisconsin Press.

Homer. (1951). The Iliad (R. Lattimore, trans.). Chicago: Univ. of Chicago Press.

Homer. (1950). The Odyssey (S. H. Butcher & A. Lang, trans.). NY: The Modern Library.

Homer-Dixon, T. (2001). *The ingenuity gap*. Toronto: Vintage Canada.

Hook, S. (1955). The hero in history. Boston: Beacon Press.

Horne, H.H. (1942). An idealistic philosophy of education. In *Proceedings of the National Society for the Study of Education*, Part I (Forty-First Yearbook), N. B. Henry (Ed.). Chicago, IL: University of Chicago Press, pp. 139-196.

Huizinga, J. (1954). *The waning of the Middle Ages*. NY: Doubleday-Anchor.

Huntington, S. P. (June 6, 1993). World politics entering a new phase, *The New York Times*, E19

Huntington, S. P. (1998). *The Clash of Civilizations (and the Remaking of World Order*. NY: Touchstone.

Huxley, J. (1957). *New wine for new bottles*. NY: Harper & Row.


Inglehart, R. and Baker, W. (2000). Modernization, cultural change and the persistence of traditional values. *American Sociological Review* 65: 19-51.

Jaeger, W. W. (1939). *Paideia: The ideals of Greek culture*, 1. NY: Oxford University Press.

James, W. (1929). *Varieties of religious experience.* NY: Longmans, Green.

Johnson, H. M. (1969). The relevance of the theory of action to historians. *Social Science Quarterly*, 2: 46-58.

Johnson, H. M. (1994). Modern organizations in the Parsonsian theory of action. In A. Farazmond, *Modern organizations: Administrative theory in contemporary society*, pp. 57 et ff. Westport, CT: Praeger.

Joseph, L.M. (1949). *Gymnastics: From the Middle Ages to the 18th century.* CIBA Symposium, 10, 5: 1030-1060.


Kahn, R. (1958). Money-muscles--and myths. In Mass leisure (E. Larrabee & R. Meyersohn, Eds.). Glencoe, IL: The Free Press.

Kaminsky, J. (1993). *A new history of educational philosophy.* Westport, CT: Greenwood Press.

Kaplan, A. (1961). *The new world of philosophy*. Boston: Houghton Mifflin.

Kateb, G. (Spring, 1965) Utopia and the good life. *Daedulus,* 92, 2:455-472.

Kaufmann, Walter. (1976). *Religions in four dimensions.* NY: Reader's Digest Press.

Kavussanu, M. & Roberts, G.C. (2001). Moral functioning in sport: An achievement goal perspective. *Journal of Sport and Exercise Psychology*, 23, 37-54.

Keating, J.W. (1964). Sportsmanship as a moral category. *Ethics*, LXXV, 1:25-35.

Keen, M. (1984). *Chivalry.* New Haven: Yale University Press.

Kennedy, J. F. (1958). (From an address by him in Detroit, Michigan while he was a U.S. Senator.)

Kennedy, P. (1987). *The rise and fall of the great powers.* NY: Random House.

Kennedy, P. (1993). *Preparing for the twenty-first century.* New York: Random House.

Kilgour, R.L. (1966). *The decline of chivalry.* Gloucester, MA: Smith.

Klapp. O.E. (1972). Heroes, villains and fools: Reflections of the American character. San Diego, CA: Aegis.

Kleinman, S. (1964). The significance of human movement--a phenomenological approach. A paper presented to the National Association of Physical Education for College Women

Conference, June 17.

Kneller, G.F. (1984). *Movements of thought in modern education.*
New York: John Wiley & Sons.

Kretchmar, R.S. (1994). *Practical philosophy of sport.*
Champaign, IL: Human Kinetics.

Krikorian, Y. H. (1944). *Naturalism and the human spirit.* NY: Columbia
University Press.


Lacroix, P. (1974). *Military and religious life in the Middle Ages
and at the period of the Renaissance.* London: Chapman & Hall.

Lauwerys, J. A. (1959) *The philosophical approach to comparative
education.* International Review of Education, V, 283-290.

LeGoff, J. (1980). *Time, work and culture in the Middle Ages.*
Chicago: Univ. of Chicago Press.

Lenk, H. (1994). Values changes and the achieving society: A socio–
philosophical perspective. In *Organization for economic cooperation and development, OECD Socieities in transition.* (pp. 81-
94)

Leonard, F. E., & Affleck G. B. (1947). *The history of physical education*
(3rd ed.). Philadelphia: Lea & Febiger.

Lewis, H. (1990) A question of values. New York, NY: Harper & Row, 1990.

Lipset. S. M. (1973). National character. In D. Koulack & D. Perlman
(Eds.), *Readings in social psychology: Focus on Canada.* Toronto:
Wiley.

London, H. (1978). The vanishing athletic hero, or whatever happened to sacrifice?
Sports, in *The New York Times*, April 23, 2.

Long, W. (2001. Athletes losing faith in hard work. *The Vancouver Sun*
(Canada), Jan. 31. E5.

Loy, J. & Hesketh, G. L. (date?). The agon motif: A prolegomenon for the study of
agonetic behavior. In *Contribution of sociology to the study of sport* (Vol. I) (K. Olin, Ed.).
Finland: Univ. of Jyvaskyla Press, pp. 31-50.

Lubin, H. (1968). The adventurer-warrior hero. In Heroes and anti-heroes (H.
Lubin, Ed.). San Francisco: Chandler.

Lumpkin, A., Stoll, S. K., & Beller, J. M. (1999). *Sport ethics:
Applications for fair play* (2nd Ed.). St. Louis: McGraw-Hill.


MacIntyre, A. (1967). Existentialism. In P. Edwards, ed., *The
Encyclopedia of Philosophy*. Vol. 3, NY: Macmillan

Magill, F.N. & Staff. (1961). *Masterworks of world philosophy*. NY:
Harper & Row.

Malina, R. M. (2001). Tracking of physical activity across the lifespan. *Research Digest (PCPFS)*, 3-14, 1-8.

March, J.G. & H.A. Simon. (1958). *Organizations*. New York: Wiley.

Marrou, H. I. (1964). *A history of education in antiquity*. Trans. George Lamb. New York: New American Library.

Marx, L. (1990). Does improved technology mean progress? In Teich, A. H. (Ed.), *Technology and the future*. NY: St. Martin's Press.

Matthew, D. (1983). *Atlas of Medieval Europe*. NY: Facts on File.

McIntosh, P. C. (1957). "Physical education in Renaissance Italy and Tudor England." In *Landmarks in the history of physical education* (J. G. Dixon, P. C. McIntosh, A. D. Munrow, & R. F. Willetts). London: Routledge & Kegan Paul.

McLean, T. (1984). *The English at play in the Middle Ages*. England: Windsor Forest. ???

McNeill W. H. (1963). *The rise of the West*. Chicago: Univ. of Chicago Press.

Meller, W. C.) (1924). *A knight's life in the days of chivalry*. London: T. Werner Lowrie.

Melnick, R. (1984). *Visions of the future*. Croton-on-Hudson, NY: Hudson Institute.

Mergen, F.. (1970). Man and his environment. *Yale Alumni Magazine*, XXXIII, 8 (May), 36-37.

Mills, C. (1826). *The history of chivalry*. Philadelphia: Carey & Lea.

Mitchell, R. J. & Leys, M. D. R. (1950). *A history of the English people*. Toronto: Longmans Green.

Monckton, O. P. (1913). *Pastimes in times past*. Philadelphia: J. P. Lippincott.

Moolenijzer, N. J. (1973). The legacy from the Middle Ages. In E. F. Zeigler (Ed. & Au.), *A history of sport to 1900*. Champaign, IL: Stipes.

Morford, W. R. & S.. J. Clark. (1976). The agon motif. In *Exercise and Sports Sciences Reviews* (Vol. 4). Santa Barbara, CA: Journal Publishing Associates, pp. 163-193.

Morgan, K. O. (Ed.). (1988). *Oxford history of Britain*, The. NY: Oxford

Morris, V. C. (1956). Physical education and the philosophy of education. *Journal of Health, Physical Education and Recreation*, (March), 21-22, 30-31.

Morrow, L. D. (1975). *Selected topics in the history of physical education in Ontario: From Dr. Egerton Ryerson to the Strathcona Trust (1844-1939)*. Ph.D. dissertation, The University of Alberta.

Muller, H. J. (1952). The uses of the past: Profiles of former societies. NY: Oxford University Press.

Muller, H. J. (1963). *The uses of the past.* NY: New American Library.

Muller, H. J. (1961). *Freedom in the ancient world.*

Muller, H. J. (1963). *Freedom in the Western world.* NY: Harper & Row.

Murray, B. G. Jr. (1972). What the ecologists can teach the economists. *The New York Times Magazine*, December 10, 38-39, 64-65, 70, 72.


Naipaul, V.S. (Oct 30, 1990). "Our Universal Civilization." The 1990 Winston Lecture, The Manhattan Institute, *New York Review of Books*, p. 20.

Naisbitt, J. (1982). *Megatrends.* New York: Warner.

Naisbitt, J. & Aburdene, P. (1990). *Megatrends* 2000. New York: Wm. Morrow.

National Association for Sport and Physical Education. (2001). The coaches code of conduct. *Strategies,* Nov.-Dec., 11.

National Geographic Society (M. Severy, Ed.). (1969). *The age of chivalry.* Washington, DC: National Geographic Society.

Naylor, D. (2002), In pursuit of level playing fields. *The Globe and Mail (Canada)*, March 9, S1.

Nevins, A. (1962). *The gateway to history.* Garden City, NY: Doubleday.

*New York Times, The.* (1970). Report by Commission on Tests of the College Entrance Examination Board, Nov. 2

Nickel, H. (1986). Games and pastimes. In J. R. Strayer (Ed.), *Dictionary of the Middle Ages.* NY: Scribner's. Pp.???

Nietzsche, F. (1958). Thus spake Zarathustra. (Transl. by A. Tille). London: J.M. Dent & Sons.

Norman, A.V.B. (1971). *The medieval soldier.* NY: Barnes & Noble.


Oldenbourgh, Z. (1948). *The world is not enough.* NY: Balantyne Books.

Olivova, V. From the arts of chivalry to gymnastics. *Canadian Journal of Sport History*, XII, 2: 29-55.

Olmert, M. (Fall 1984). Chaucer's little lotteries: The literary use of a medieval game. *Arete: Journal of Sport Literature* II, 1:171-182.

Olson, G. (1980). *Reading as recreation in the later Middle Ages.* Ithaca, NY: Cornell Univ. Press.

Oldenbourgh, Z. (1948). The world is not enough. NY: Balantyne Books.

Osterhoudt, R G. (2006). *Sport as a form of human fulfillment: An organic philosophy of sport history*. (Vol. I and II).Victoria, Canada: Trafford.

Osterhoudt, R. G. (2010). Personal correspondence, April 9. (For further analysis. See his "Concluding Postscript" (pp. 723-726) in Osterhoudt's *Sport as a form of human fulfillmentÚ An organic philosophy of sport history* (Victoria, BC, Canada, 2006)


Painter, S. (1962). *French chivalry*. Baltimore: Johns Hopkins Press.

Paton, G. A. (1975). The historical background and present status of Canadian physical education. In E .F. Zeigler (Ed.), *A history of physical education and sport in the United States and Canada* (pp. 441-443). Champaign, IL: Stipes.

Perry, R. B. (1955). *Present philosophical tendencies*. NY: George Braziller.

Platt, C. (1979). *The atlas of medieval man*. NY: St. Martin's Press.

Plumb, J. H. (1961). *Renaissance profiles*. NY: Harper & Row.

Priest, R. F., Krause, J. V., & Beach, J. (1999). Four-year changes in college athletes' ethical value choices in sports situations. *Research Quarterly for Exercise and Sport, 70*, 1, 170-178.

*Province, The* (Vancouver, Canada) (2000). Drug allegations rock sports world. July 3, A2.


Rand, A. (1960). *The romantic manifesto*. New York: World Publishing Co.

Random House dictionary of the English language (1967) (Jess Stein, Ed.). NY: Random House.

Rees-Mogg, W. (1988). The decline of the Olympics into physical and moral squalor. *Coaching Focus*, 8 (1988),

Reisner, E. H. (1925). *Nationalism and education since 1789*. New York: Macmillan.

Renson, R. (1976). *The Flemish Archery Guilds: From defense mechanisms to sports institutions*. Mainz: Dokumente des V HISPA Kongresses, pp. 135-139.

Riesman, D. (1954). The themes of heroism and weakness in the structure of Freud's thought. In *Selected Essays from Individualism Reconsidered*. Garden City, NY: Doubleday.

Roberts, J. M. (1993). *A short history of the world*. NY: Oxford University Press.

Rorty, R. (1997) *Achieving our country*. Cambridge, MA: Harvard University Press

Rowling, M. (1968). *Everyday life in medieval times*. NY: Dorset.

Royce, J. R. (1964). Paths to knowledge. In *The encapsulated man* Princeton, NJ: Van Nostrand.

Rudd, A., Stoll, S .K., & Beller, J. M. (1999). Measuring moral and social character among a group of Division 1A college athletes, non-athletes, and ROTC military students. *Research Quarterly for Exercise and Sport*, 70 (Suppl. 1), 127.

Rudorff, R. (1974). *Knights and the age of chivalry*. NY: Viking Press.

Russell, B. (1959). *Wisdom of the West*. London: Rathbone Books

Sage, G. H. (1988, October). "Sports participation as a builder of character?" *The World and I*, Vol. 3, 629-641.

Sage, G. H. (1998). Sports participation as a builder of character? *The World and I*, 3, 629-641.

Scarre, C. (1993). *Smithsonian timelines of the ancient world*. London: Dorling Kindersly.

Schein, S. L. (1984). *The mortal hero*. Berkeley, CA: Univ. of California Press.

Schlesinger, A. M. (1998). (Rev. & Enl.).*The disuniting of America*. NY: W.W. Norton.

Schopenhauer, A. (1946). The world as will and idea. In F. N. Magill (Ed.), *Master-works of philosophy*. NY: Doubleday.

Schrodt. B. Sports of the Byzantine Empire, *The Journal of Sport History*, VIII, 3: 40-59.

Sellars, R. W. (1932). *The philosophy of physical realism*. NY: Macmillan.

Sigerist, H. E. (1956). *Landmarks in the history of hygiene*. London: Oxford University Press.

Silvers, S. (1984). Letter to the Editor. *Sports Illustrated*, October 29.

Simpson, G. G. (1949). *The meaning of evolution*. New Haven & London: Yale University Press.

Skaset, H. B., Email correspondence. May 14, 2002.

Smith, H. (1831). *Festivals, games, and amusements*. London: Colburn & Bentley.

Spears, B. & Swanson, R. (1988). *History of sport and physical education in the United States*. Dubuque, IA: Championship Books.

Spencer-Kraus, P. (1969). The application of "linguistic phenomenology" to the philosophy of physical education and sport. M. A. thesis, University of Illinois, U-C.

Spiegelberg, H. (1976). *The phenomenological movement: An introduction*. (Vol. 1, Rev. Ed.). The Hague: Nijhoff.

Stark, S. D. (1987). Entertainment, in *The New York Times*, February 22, 19.

Steinhaus, A. H. (1952). Principal principles of physical education.
In *Proceedings of the College Physical Education Association.*
Washington, DC: AAHPER, pp. 5-11.

Stoll, S. K. & Beller, J. M. (1998). *Sport as education: On the edge.* NY: Columbia
University Teachers College

Strohmeyer, H. (1977). Physical education of the princes in the late
Middle Ages as depicted by two works of the Styrian Abbot,
Engelbert of Admont (1250-1331 A.D.). *Canadian Journal of Sport
and Physical Education*, 1: 38-48.


Ten events that shook the world between 1984 and 1994. (Special
Report). *Utne Reader*, 62 (March/April 1994): 58-74

Thomas, K. (Dec. 1964). Work and leisure in pre-industrial society.
*Past and present*, 29: 50-62.

Tibbetts, J. (2002). Spend more on popular sports, Canadians say,
*National Post* (Canada), A8, April 15.

Tierney, B. (1974). *The Middle Ages, Vol. II: Readings in Medieval
History*. (2nd Ed.). NY: Knopf.

Toffler, A. (1970). *Future shock.* New York: Random House.

Toffler, A. (1980). *The third wave*. New York: Bantam Books.

Toynbee, A. J. (1947). *A study of history.* NY: Oxford University Press.

Treharne, R.F. & Fullard, H. (Eds.). (1961). *Muir's New School Atlas
of Universal History*. (21st Ed.). Barnes & Noble.

Tuchman, B.W. (1978). *A distant mirrow: The calamitous 14th century*.
NY: Knopf.


Ueberhorst, H. (Ed.) (1978). *Geschichte der Leibesuebungen (*Vol. 2).
Berlin: Verlag Bartels & Wernitz.

Ullman, W. (1965). *A history of political thought: The Middle Ages.*
Baltimore, MD: Penguin.


Van Dalen, D. B. (1973). The idea of history of physical education
during the Middle Ages and Renaissance. In E.F. Zeigler (Ed. & Au.),
*A history of sport and physical education to 1900 (*pp. 217-224).
Champaign, IL: Stipes.

Van Dalen, D. B., E. D. Mitchell, & B. L. Bennett. (1953). *A world
history of physical education*. (1st Ed.). Englewood Cliffs, NJ:
Prentice-Hall. (A second edition was also published.)

VanderZwaag, H. J. (1982) Background, meaning, and significance. In
E. F. Zeigler, (Ed. & Au.). *Physical education and sport: An Introduction* (p. 54).

Philadelphia: Lea & Febiger.

Veblen, T. (1899). The theory of the leisure class. NY: Macmillan.

Von Neumann, J. & Morgenstern, O. (1947). *The theory of games and economic behavior.* (2nd ed.). Princeton: Princeton University Press.


Wallis, D. (2002). Annals of Olympics filled with dubious decisions. *National Post* (Canada), Feb. 16, B2.

Warre-Cornish, F. (1901). *Chivalry.* London: Swan Sonnenschein.

Wecter, D. (1941). *The hero in America: A chronicle of hero worship.* NY: Charles Scribner's Sons.

Weiner, J. (Jan.-Feb. 2000). Why our obsession has ruined the game; and how we can save it. *Utne Reader,* 97, 48-50.

Weinstein, M. (1991). Critical thinking and the post-modern challenge to educational practice. *Inquiry: Critical Thinking Across the Disciplines,* 7:1, 1,14.

Welzel, C., Inglehart, R., & Klingerman, H–D. (2003). The theory of human development: A cross-cultural analysis." *European Journal of Political Research* 42(3): 341-79.

White, M. (1962). *The age of analysis.* Boston: Houghton Mifflin.

White, L. (1962). *Medieval technology and social change.* London: Oxford University Press.

Wilcox, R. C. (1991). Sport and national character: An empirical analysis. *Journal of Comparative Physical Education and Sport.*, XIII(1), 3-27.

Wild, J. Education and human society: A realistic view. In N.B. Henry (Ed.), *Modern philosophies and education* (Part I). (1955). Chicago, Univ. of Chicago Press.

Williams, J. Paul. (1952). *What Americans believe and how they worship.* New York: Harper & Row.

Windelband, W. (1901). *A history of philosophy.* (Vol. I and II). (Rev. Ed.). NY: Harper & Row.

Wood, M. (1987). *In search of the Dark Ages.* NY: Facts on File.

Woodward, W.H. (1905). *Vittorino da Feltre and other humanist educators.* Cambridge University Press. (Reprinted from 1897 ed.).

Woody, T. (1949). *Life and education in early societies.* New York: Macmillan.


Zeigler, E. F. (1951). *A history of undergraduate professional preparation in physical education in the United States, 1861-1948.* Eugene, OR: Oregon Microfiche.

Zeigler, E. F. (1964). *Philosophical foundations for physical, health, and recreation education.* Englewood Cliffs, NJ: Prentice-Hall.

Zeigler, E. F. (1965). *A brief introduction to the philosophy of religion.* Champaign, IL: Stipes.

Zeigler, E. F. (1968). *Problems in the history and philosophy of physical education and sport.* Englewood Cliffs, NJ: Prentice-Hall.

Zeigler, E. F. (Ed. & Au.). (1973). *A history of sport and physical education to 1900.* Champaign, IL: Stipes.

Zeigler, E. F. (1975). Historical perspective on contrasting philosophies of professional preparation for physical education in the United States. In *Personalizing physical education and sport philosophy* (pp. 325-347). Champaign, IL: Stipes.

Zeigler, E. F. (Ed. & author). (1975). *A history of physical education and sport in the United States and Canada.* Champaign, IL: Stipes.

Zeigler, E. F. (1977a). *Physical education and sport philosophy.* Englewood Cliffs, NJ: Prentice-Hall.

Zeigler, E. F. (1977b). Philosophical perspective on the future of physical education and sport. In R. Welsh (Ed.), *Physical education: A view toward the future* (pp. 36-61). Saint Louis: C.V. Mosby.

Zeigler, E. F. (1979). *Issues in North American Physical Education and Sport.* Washington, DC: AAHPERD.

Zeigler, E. F. and Bowie, G. W. (1983).*Management competency development in physical education and sport.* Philadelphia: Lea & Febiger.

Zeigler, E .F. (1984). Ethics and morality in sport and physical education. Champaign, IL: Stipes.

Zeigler, E. F. (1986). *Assessing Sport and Physical Education: Diagnosis and Projection* \ Champaign, IL: Stipes.

Zeigler, E. F. (1987). Babe Ruth or Lou Gehrig: A United States' dilemma. *The Physical Educator,* 44, 2.:325-329.

Zeigler, E. F. (Ed. & author). (1988). *A history of physical education and sport* (Rev. ed.). Champaign, IL: Stipes.

Zeigler, E. F. (1988). Physical education and sport in the Middle Ages. In

Zeigler, E. F. (1989). *Sport and physical education philosophy.* Dubuque, IA: Benchmark/W.C. Brown.

Zeigler, E. F. (1990*). Sport and Physical Education: Past, Present, Future.* Champaign, IL: Stipes, 1991).

Zeigler, E. F. (May 1993). Chivalry's influence on sport and physical training in Medieval Europe. *Canadian Journal of History of Sport,* XXIV, 1:1-17.

Zeigler, E. F. (1994) *Critical Thinking for the Professions: Health, Sport and Physical Education, Recreation, and Dance.* Champaign IL: Stipes Publishing L.L.C.

Zeigler, E. F. (ed. & au.). (1994) *Physical education and kinesiology in North America: Professional and scholarly foundations.* Champaign, IL: Stipes Publishing Co.

Zeigler, E. F. (Sept.,1994). Physical education's "principal principles". *JOPERD*, 54, 4-5. (This was published, also, in the *CAHPERD Journal*, Spring, 1995, Vol. 61, No. 1: 20-21.

Zeigler, E. F. (1996). Historical perspective on "quality of life": Genes. memes, and physical activity. *Quest*, 48, 246-263.

Zeigler, E. F. (2003). *Socio-Cultural Foundations of Physical Education and Educational Sport.* Aachen, Germany: Meyer & Meyer Sport.

Zeigler, E. F. (2005). *History and Status of American Physical Education and Educational Sport.* Victoria, Canada: Trafford.

Zeigler, E. F. (Spring, 2006b) What the field of physical (activity) education should do in the immediate future. *The Journal of the International Council of Health, Physical Education, Recreation, Sport, and Dance,* XLII, 2:35-39. (This article was also published in 2006 in the *ICHPERSD Journal of Research in Health, Physical Education, Recreation, Sport, and Dance.*)

Zeigler, E. F. (2007). *Applied Ethics for Sport and Physical Activity Professionals.* Victoria, Canada: Trafford.

Zeigler, E. F. (2009). *Sport and Physical Activity in Human History: A Persistent Problems Approach.* Bloomington, IN: Trafford.

Zeigler, E. F. (Ed. & Au.). (2009). *An Anthology of American Physical Education and Sport History.* Bloomington, IN: Trafford, 2009.

Zeigler, E. F. (Ed. & Au.) (2009). *International & Comparative Physical Education and Sport.* Bloomington, IN: Trafford

Zeigler, E. F. (2010). *The American Crisis in Physical Activity Education: Confusing Winning at Sport With Total Fitness for All.* Bloomington, IN: Trafford, 2009.

Zeigler, E. F. (2010). *Philosophy of Physical Activity Education (including Sport).* Bloomington, IN: Trafford.

Zeigler, E. F. (2010). *Management Theory and Practice in Physical Activity Education (including Athletics).* Bloomington, IN: Trafford.

Zeldin, T. (1994). *An intimate history of humanity.* NY: HarperCollins.

Zetterberg, H. L. (1965). *On theory and verification in sociology.* Totowa, NJ: The Bedminster Press.

# Appendix A
## Determining Values through Philosophic Self-Evaluation in Life, Education, and Developmental Physical Activity

## Introduction

What follows is the latest version of a philosophic, self-evaluation checklist designed for men and women who are specializing in the field of physical activity education in exercise, sport, and physical recreation. I developed this checklist originally in the early 1950s, but it has been revised and updated regularly over the years to reflect all of the positions, tendencies, and stances described below. By employing this instructional device carefully and honestly--while appreciating the subjectivity of an instrument such as this--aspiring professionals will be able to determine quite accurately their philosophy of life (including an ethical position), their philosophy of education, and their philosophy of developmental physical activity in exercise and sport insofar as its possible meaning and significance in people's lives are concerned. (Additional subsections not included here have been developed for the professions of health and safety education and recreation/recreation education as well.)

Before examining himself or herself, we suggest that each person study briefly the Freedom-Constraint Spectrum below. (You will be asked to do this again after you have completed the professional, self-evaluation, philosophic checklist and have evaluated your personal position.) Keep in mind that the primary criterion on which this is based is the concept of 'personal freedom' in contrast to 'personal constraint'. Herbert J. Muller's definition of freedom (1954) calls it "the condition of being able to choose and to carry out purposes" in one's personal living pattern.

Within our social environment, the words "progressive" or "liberal" and "conservative" or "traditional" have historically related to policies favoring individual freedom and policies favoring adherence to tradition, respectively. For this reason, the more traditional positions or stances are shown to the right on the spectrum, and the more progressive ones are shown to the left. The analytic approach to doing philosophy is included in the checklist, but it is not shown on the spectrum because it has indeed become "philosophy in a new key." The earlier, mainstream positions in educational philosophy are indicated in parentheses on the figure below. Other pertinent definitions of positions on the freedom-constraint spectrum are offered immediately below the figure itself.

## Figure 1
## The Freedom-Constraint Spectrum

Eclecticism*

Existentialism**            Traditional
(atheistic, agnostic,      or  (Idealism)
or theistic)
Somewhat Progressive      Traditional
(Reconstructionism)       (Naturalistic Realism)

Progressive              Traditional
(Pragmatic Naturalism)      Rational Humanism)

Strongly Progressive       Strongly Traditional
(Romantic Naturalism)       Scholastic Realism)

ANARCHY                  DICTATORSHIP

"the left"                  "the right"

*Analytic*--a philosophic outlook, actually with ancient origins, that moved ahead strongly in the twentieth century. The assumption here has been that our ordinary language has many defects that need to be corrected. There is concern also with conceptual analysis. Another objective is "the rational reconstruction of the language of science" (Abraham Kaplan). Basically, the preoccupation is with analysis as opposed to philosophical system-building.

* The so-called eclectic approach is placed in the center because it assumes that the person evaluating himself or herself has selected several positions on opposite sides of the spectrum. Most would argue that eclecticism is philosophically indefensible, while some believe that "patterned eclecticism" (or "reasoned incoherence" as this position has been called) represents a stance which most of us hold.

** Existentialistic--a permeating influence rather than a full-blown philosophical position. Keep in mind that there are those with either an atheistic, agnostic, or theistic orientation. This position has been shown slightly to the left of center because within this stance(tendency) there is a strong emphasis on individual freedom of choice.

Instructions:  Read the statements below carefully, section by section, and indicate by an X the statement in each section that seems closest to your own personal belief.

Check your answers only after all FIVE sections have been completed.  Then complete the summarizing tally on the answer page.  Take note of apparent inconsistencies in your overall position.  Finally, return to the freedom-constraint spectrum above to discover your "location" whether in the center--or to the right or left.

Note:  Many of the words, terms, phrases, etc. have been obtained from the work of philosophers, educational philosophers, and sport and physical education philosophers, living or deceased. I am most grateful for this assistance, but in the final analysis decided to leave them unidentified so as not to prejudice the person taking the test. In this self-evaluation check list, sections relating to the allied professions (e.g., recreation) have been deliberately omitted, but they are available upon request.

Keep in mind that we are not seeking to make the case that, for example, a position taken under (say) Category I will result by logical deduction in a comparable position being taken in a following category either within the education or sport and physical education categories. Nevertheless, positions taken in these latter categories should, to be consistent, probably be grounded on philosophical presuppositions stated earlier.

## Category I
## THE NATURE OF REALITY (METAPHYSICS)

A. _____  Experience and nature constitute both the form and also the content of the entire universe. There is no such thing as a pre-established order of affairs in the world. Reality is evolving, and humanity appears to be a most important manifestation of the natural process. The impact of cultural forces upon people is fundamental, and every effort should be made to understand them as we strive to build the best type of a group-centered culture. In other words, the structure of cultural reality should be our foremost concern. Cultural determinants have shaped human history, and a crucial stage has now been reached in the development of life on the planet. Our efforts must now be focused on the building of a world culture.

B. _____  I believe that the metaphysical and normative types of philosophizing have lost their basis for justification in the twentieth century. Their presumed wisdom has not been able to withstand the rigor of careful analysis. Sound theory is available to humankind through the application of scientific method to problem-solving. So what is the exact nature of philosophy? Who is in a position to answer the ultimate questions about the nature of reality? The scientist is, of course, and the philosopher must become the servant of science through conceptual analysis and the rational reconstruction of language. Accordingly the philosopher must resign himself or herself to dealing with important, but lesser, questions than the origin of the universe and the nature of the human being--and what implications this might have for everyday conduct.

C. _____  The world of men and women is a human one, and it is from the context of this human world that all the abstractions of science derive their meaning ultimately. There is the world of

227

material objects that extends in mathematical space with only quantitative and measurable properties, but we humans are first and foremost "concrete involvements" within the world. Existence precedes essence, and it is up to men and women to decide their own fate. This presumably makes the human different from all other creatures on earth. It appears true that people can actually transform life's present condition, and thus the future may well stand open to these unusual beings.

D. _____ Nature is an emergent evolution, and the human's frame of reality is limited to nature as it functions. The world is characterized by activity and change. Rational man and woman have developed through organic evolution over millions of years, and the world is yet incomplete--a reality that is constantly undergoing change because of a theory of emergent novelty that appears to be operating within the universe. People enjoy true freedom of will. This freedom is achieved through continuous and developmental learning from experience.

E. _____ Mind as experience by all people is basic and real. The entire universe is mind essentially. The human is more than just a body; people possess souls, and such possession makes them of a higher order than all other creatures on earth. The order of the world is due to the manifestation in space and time of an eternal and spiritual reality. The individual is simply part of the whole. It is therefore a person's duty to learn as much about the Absolute as possible. Within this position there is divided opinion regarding the problem of monism or pluralism (one force or more than one force). The individual person has freedom to determine which way he or she will go in life. The individual can relate to the moral law in the universe, or else he or she can turn against it.

## Category II
## ETHICS AND MORALITY (Axiology/Values)

A. _____ The source of all human experience lies in the regularities of the universe. Things don't just happen; they happen because many interrelated forces make them occur in a particular way. Humans in this environment are confronted by one reality only--that which we perceive is it! The "life of reason" is extremely important, a position that emanates originally from Aristotle who placed intellectual virtues above moral virtues in his hierarchy. Many holding this stance believe that all elements of nature, including people, are inextricably linked together in an endless chain of causes and effects. Thus, they accept a sort of ethical determinism--i.e., what people are morally is determined by response patterns imprinted in their being by both heredity and environment. A large number in the world carry this fundamental position still further by adding a theological component; for them the highest good is ultimate union with God, the Creator, who is responsible for teleological and supernatural reality. As a creature of God, human goodness is reached by the spirituality of the form attained as the individual achieves emancipation from the material (or the corporeal). The belief is that a person's being contains potential energy that may be guided or directed toward God or away from Him; thus, what the individual does in the final analysis determines whether such action will be regarded as right or wrong.

B. _____ There should be no distinction between moral goods and natural goods. There has been a facts/values dualism in existence, and this should be eradicated as soon as possible by the use of scientific method applied to ethical situations. Thus, we should employ reflective thinking to obtain the ideas that will function as tentative solutions for the solving of life's concrete problems. Those ideas can serve as hypotheses to be tested in life experimentally. If the ideas work in solving problematic situations, they become true. In this way we have empirical verification of hypotheses tending to bring theory and practice into a closer union. When we achieve agreement in factual belief, agreement in attitudes about this subject should soon follow. In this way science can ultimately bring about complete agreement on factual belief or knowledge about human behavior. Thus there will be a continuous adaptation of values to the culture's changing needs that will in turn effect the directed reconstruction of all social institutions.

C. _____ The problems of ethics should be resolved quite differently than they have throughout most of history. Ethics cannot be resolved completely through the application of scientific method, although an ethical dispute must be on a factual level--i.e., factual statements must be distinguished from value statements. Ethics should be normative in the sense that we have moral standards. However, this is a difficult task because the term "good" appears to be indefinable. The terms used to define or explain ethical standards or norms should be analyzed logically in a careful manner. Social scientists should be enlisted to help in the determination of the validity of factual statements, as well as in the analysis of conflicting attitudes as progress is determined. Ethical dilemmas in modern life can be resolved through the combined efforts of the philosophical moralist and the scientist. The resultant beliefs may in time change people's attitudes. Basically, the task is to establish a hierarchy of reasons with a moral basis.

D. _____ Good and bad, and rightness and wrongness, are relative and vary according to the situation or culture involved (i.e., the needs of a situation are there and then in that society or culture). Each ethical decision is highly individual, initially at least, since every situation has its particularity. The free, authentic individual decides to accept responsibility when he or she responds to a human situation and seeks to answer the need of an animal, person, or group. How does the "witness react to the world?" Guidance in the making of an ethical decision may come either from "outside," from intuition, from one's own conscience, from reason, from empirical investigation, etc. Thus it can be argued that there are no absolutely valid ethical principles or universal laws.

E. _____ Ethics and morality are based on cosmic laws, and we are good if we figure out how to share actively in them. If we have problems of moral conduct, we have merely to turn to the Lord's commandments for solutions to all moral problems. Yet there is nothing deterministic here, because the individual himself or herself has an active role to play in determining which ethical actions will bring him or her into closer unity with the supreme Self. However, the fact of the matter is that God is both the source and the goal of the values for which we strive in our everyday lives. In this approach the presence of evil in the world is recognized as a real human experience to be met and conquered. The additional emphasis here is on logical argument to counter the ever-present threat of the philosophy of science. This is countered by the argument that there is unassailable moral law inherent in the Universe that presents people with obligations to duty (e.g., honesty is a good that is universal).

F. _____ Our social environment is inextricably related to the many struggles of peoples for improvement of the quality of life--how to place more good in our lives than bad, so to speak. We are opposed to any theory that delineates values as absolute and separates them from everyday striving within a social milieu. Actually the truth of values can be determined by established principles of evidence. In an effort to achieve worldwide consensus on any and all values, our stated positions on issues and controversial matters must necessarily be criticized in public forums. Cultural realities that affect values should be re-oriented through the achievement of agreed-upon purposes (i.e., through social consensus and social-self-realization on a worldwide basis). The goal, then, is to move toward a comprehensive pattern of values that provides both flexibility and variety. This should be accompanied by sufficient freedom to allow the individual to achieve individual and social values in his or her life. However, we must not forget that the majority does rule in evolving democracies, and at times wrong decisions are made. Keeping in mind that the concept of 'democracy' will prevail only to the extent that "enlightened" decisions are made, we must guarantee the ever-present role of the critical minority as it seeks to alter any consensus established. A myth of utopian vision should guide our efforts as we strive toward the achievement of truly human ethical values in the life experiences of all our citizens.

## Category III
## EDUCATIONAL AIMS AND OBJECTIVES

A. _____ Socialization of the child has become equally as important as his or her intellectual development as a key educational aim in this century. There should be concern, however, because many educational philosophers seem to assume the position that children are to be fashioned so that they will conform to a prior notion of what they should be. Even the progressivists seem to have failed in their effort to help the learner "posture himself or herself." If it does become possible to get general agreement on a set of fundamental dispositions to be formed, should the criterion employed for such evaluation be a public one (rather than personal and private)? Education should seek to "awaken awareness" in the learner--awareness of the person as a single subjectivity in the world. Increased emphasis is needed on the arts and social sciences, and the student should freely and creatively choose his or her own pattern of education.

B. _____ Social-self-realization is the supreme value in education. The realization of this ideal is most important for the individual in the social setting--a world culture. Positive ideals should be molded toward the evolving democratic ideal by a general education which is group-centered and in which the majority determines the acceptable goals. However, once that majority opinion is determined, all are obligated to conform until such majority opinion can be reversed (the doctrine of "defensible partiality"). Nevertheless, education by means of "hidden coercion" is to be scrupulously avoided. Learning itself is explained by the organismic principle of functional psychology. Social intelligence acquired teaches people to control and direct their urges as they concur with or attempt to modify cultural purposes.

C. _____ The concept of 'education' has become much more complex that was ever realized before. Because of the various meanings of the term "education," talking about educational aims and objectives is almost a hopeless task unless a myriad of qualifications is used for clarification. The term ("education") has now become what is called a "family-resemblance" term in philosophy. Thus we need to qualify our meaning to explain to the listener whetrher we mean (1) the subject-matter; (2) the activity of education carried on by teachers; (3) the process of being educated (or learning) that is occurring; (4) the result, actual oir intended, or No.2 and No.3 Immediately above taking place through the employment of that which comprises No.1 above; (5) the discipline, or field of enquiry and investigation; and (6) the profession whose members are involved professionally with all of the aspects of education described above. With this understanding, it is then possible to make some determination about which specific objectives the profession of education should strive for as it moves in the direction of the achievement of long range aims.

D. _____ The general aim of education is more education. Education in the broadest sense can be nothing else than the changes made in human beings by their experience. Participation by students in the formation of aims and objectives is absolutely essential to generate the all-important desired interest required for the finest educational process to occur. Social efficiency (i.e., societal socialization) can well be considered the general aim of education. Pupil growth is a paramount goal. This means that the individual is placed at the center of the educational experience.

E. _____ A philosophy which holds that the aim of education is the acquisition of verified knowledge of the environment; which recognizes the value of content as well as the activities involved; and which takes into account the external determinants of human behavior. Education is the acquisition of the art of the utilization of knowledge. The primary task of education is to transmit knowledge, knowledge without which civilization could not continue to flourish. Whatever people have discovered to be true because it conforms to reality should be handed down to future generations as the social or cultural tradition. Some holding this philosophy believe that the good life emanates from cooperation with God's grace, and believe further that the development of the Christian virtues is obviously of greater worth than learning or anything else.

F. _____ Through education the developing organism becomes what it latently is. All education may be said to have a religious significance, the meaning of which is that there is a "moral imperative" on education. As the person's mind strives to realize itself, there is the possibility of the Absolute within the individual mind. Education should aid the child to adjust to the basic realities (the spiritual ideals of truth, beauty, and goodness) that the history of the race has furnished us. The basic values of human living are health, character, social justice, skill, art, love, knowledge, philosophy, and religion.

## Category IV
## THE EDUCATIVE PROCESS
### (Epistemology)

A. _____ Understanding the nature of knowledge will clarify the nature of reality. Nature is the medium by which the Absolute communicates to us. Basically, knowledge comes only from the mind, a mind which must offer and receive ideas. Mind and matter are qualitatively different. A finite mind emanates through heredity from another finite mind. Thought is the standard by which all else in the world is judged. An individual attains truth for himself or herself by examining the wisdom of the past through his or her own mind. Reality, viewed in this way, is a system of logic and order that has been established by the Universal Mind. Experimental testing helps to determine what the truth really is.

B. _____ The child experiences an "awareness of being" in his/her subjective life about the time of puberty--and is never the same thereafter. The young person truly becomes aware of his or her own existence, and the fact that there is now a responsibility for one's own conduct. After this point in life, education must be an "act of discovery" to be truly effective. Somehow the teacher should help the young person to become involved personally with his or her education, and also with the world situation in which such an education is taking place. Objective or subjective knowledge should be personally selected and 'appropriated" by the youth unto himself or herself, or else it will be relatively meaningless in that particular life. Thus it matters not whether logic, scientific evidence, sense perception, intuition, or revelation is claimed as the basis og knowledge acquisition, no learning will take place for that individual self until the child or young person decides that such learning is "true" for him or her in that person's life. Therefore the young person knows when he or she knows!

C. _____ Knowledge is the result of a process of thought with a useful purpose. Truth is not only to be tested by its correspondence with reality, but also by its practical results. Knowledge is earned through experience and is an instrument of verification. Mind has evolved in the natural order as a more flexible means whereby people adapt themselves to the world. Learning takes place when interest and effort unite to produce the desired result. A psychological order of learning (problem-solving as explained through scientific method) is ultimately more useful (productive?) than a logical arrangement (proceeding from the simple fact to the complex conclusion). However, we shouldn't forget that there is always a social context to learning, and the curriculum itself should be adapted to the particular society for which it is intended.

D. _____ Concern with the educative process should begin with an understanding of the terms that are typically employed for discussion purposes within any educational program. The basic assumption is that these terms are usually employed loosely and often improperly. For example, to be precise we should be explaining that a student is offered educational experiences in a classroom and/or laboratory setting. Through the employment of various types and techniques of instructional methodology (e.g., lectures), he or she hears facts, increases the scope of information and/or knowledge, and learns to comprehend and interpret the material (understanding). Possessing various kinds and amounts of ability or aptitude, students    gradually develop competencies and a certain degree or level of skill. It is hoped that certain appreciations about the worth of the individual student's experiences will be developed, and that he or she will form certain attitudes about familial, societal, and professional life that lie ahead. Finally, societal

232

values and norms, along with other social influences, will help educators, fulfilling role within their collectivities and sub–collectivities, determine the best methods (with accompanying experimentation, of course) of achieving socially acceptable educational goals.

E. \_\_\_\_ An organismic approach to the learning process is basic. Thought cannot be independent of certain aspects of the organism. This is because thought is related integrally with emotional and muscular functions. The person's mind enables him or her to cope with the problems of human life in a social environment within a physical world. Social intelligence is actually closely related to scientific method. Certain operational concepts, inseparable from metaphysics and axiology (beliefs about reality and values), focus on the reflective thought, problem-solving, and social consensus necessary for the gradual transformation of the culture.

F. \_\_\_\_ There are two major learning (epistemological) theories of knowledge in this philosophical stance. One states that the aim of knowledge is to bring into awareness the object as it really is. The other emphasizes that objects are "represented" in the human's consciousness, not "presented." Students should develop habits and skills involved with acquiring knowledge, with using knowledge practically to meet life's problems, and with realizing the enjoyment that life offers. A second variation of learning theory (epistemological belief) here indicates that the child develops his or her intellect by employing reason to learn a subject. The principal educational aims proceeding hand in hand with learning theory here would be the same for all people at all times in all places. Others with a more religious orientation holding this position, basically add to this stance that education is the process by which people seek to link themselves ultimate with their Creator.

## Category V
## VALUES IN SPECIALIZED FIELD
### (Developmental Physical Activity in Exercise and Sport)

A. \_\_\_\_ I believe in the concept of 'total fitness' which implies an educational design directed toward the individual's self-realization as a social being. In our field there should be an opportunity for selection of a wide variety of useful activities. Instruction in human motor performance relating to sport, exercise, dance, and play is necessary to provide a sufficient amount of "physical" fitness activity. The introduction of dance, music, and art into physical education can contribute to the person's creative expression. Intramural sports and voluntary physical recreational activities should be stressed. This applies especially to team competitions with particular stress on cooperation and the promotion of friendly competition. Extramural sport competition should be introduced when there is a need. Striving for excellence is important, but it is vital that materialistic influences should be kept out of the educational program. In today's increasingly stressful environment, relaxation techniques should have a place too, as should the concept of 'education for leisure.'

B. \_\_\_\_ I believe that the field of developmental physical activity in exercise and sport should strive to fulfill a role in the general education pattern of the arts and sciences. The goal is total fitness, not only physical fitness, with a balance between activities emphasizing competition and cooperation. The concepts of 'universal man' and 'universal woman' are paramount, but we must allow the individual to choose his or her sport, exercise, and dance activities for himself or herself based on knowledge of self and what knowledge and/or skills he or she would like to possess. We should help the child who is "authentically eccentric" feel at home in the sport and physical education program. It is also important that we find ways for youth to commit themselves to values and people. A person should be able (and permitted) to select developmental physical activity according to the values which he or she wishes to derive from it. This is often difficult in our society today because of the extreme overemphasis placed on winning--being "Number 1!" Finally, creative movement activities such as modern dance should be stressed, also.

C. \_\_\_\_ I believe that education "of the physical" should have primary emphasis in our field. I am concerned with the development of physical vigor, and such development should have priority over the recreational aspects of sport and physical education. Many people, who hold the same educational philosophy as I do, recommend that all students in public schools should have a daily period designed to strengthen their muscles and develop their bodily coordination and circulo-respiratory endurance. Developmental physical activity must, of course, yield precedence to intellectual education. I give qualified approval to interscholastic, intercollegiate, and inter-university athletics, since they do help with the learning of sportsmanship and desirable social conduct if properly carried out. However, all these objectives, with the possible exception of physical training, are definitely extra-curricular and not part of what we call the regular educational curriculum.

D. \_\_\_\_ I am much more interested in promoting the concept of 'total fitness' rather than physical fitness alone. I believe that sport and physical education should be considered an integral subject in the curriculum. Students should have the opportunity to select a wide variety of useful activities, many of which should help to develop "social intelligence." The activities offered should bring what are considered as natural impulses into play. To me, developmental physical activity classes and intramural-recreational sports are much more important to the large majority of students than highly competitive athletics offered at considerable expense for the few. Thus sport and physical education for the "normal" or "special" young man or woman deserves priority if conflict arises over budgetary allotment, staff availability, and facility use. However, I can still give full support to "educational" competitive sport, because such individual, dual, and/or team activities can provide vital educational experiences for young people if properly conducted.

E. \_\_\_\_ I believe that there is a radical, logically fundamental difference between statements of what is the case and statements of what ought to be the case. When people express their beliefs about developmental physical activity in exercise and sport, their disagreements can be resolved in principle. However, it is logical also that there can be sharing of beliefs (facts, knowledge) with radical disagreement in attitudes. In a democracy, for example, we can conceivably agree on the fact that jogging (or bicycling, swimming, walking, etc.) brings about certain circulo-respiratory changes, but we can't force people to get actively involved or even to hold a favorable attitude toward such activity. We can demonstrate tenable theory about such physical involvement, therefore, but we cannot prove that a certain attitude toward such activity is the correct one. Thus I may accept evidence that vigorous sport, dance, exercise, and play can bring about certain effects or changes in the organism, but my own attitude and subsequent regular involvement--the values in it for me--is the result of a commitment rather than a prediction.

F. \_\_\_\_ I am extremely interested in individual personality development. I believe in education "of the physical," and yet I believe in education "though the physical" as well. Accordingly, I see sport and physical education as important, but also occupying a lower rung on the educational ladder. I believe that desirable objectives for sport and physical education would include the development of responsible citizenship and group participation. In competitive sport I believe that the transfer of training theory is in operation in connection with the development of desirable personality traits (or undesirable traits if the leadership is poor). Participation in highly competitive sport should always serve as a means to a desirable end.

**Note**: Appreciation should be expressed at this point to the many people from whose work phrases and very short quotations were taken for inclusion in the checklist. Inclusion of their names at those particular points in the checklist did not seem advisable, inasmuch as the particular position or stance may have been instantly recognized.

Answers:  Read only after all five questions have been completed.
Record your answer to each part of the checklist on the
summarizing tally form below.

## I.  The Nature of Reality (Metaphysics)

    a.  Somewhat Progressive
    b.  Analytic (Analytic Philosophy)
    c.  Existentialistic (atheistic, agnostic, or theistic)
    d.  Progressive (Pragmatic Naturalism; Ethical Naturalism)
    e.  Traditional (Philosophic Idealism)
    f.  Traditional (Philosophic Realism, with elements of Naturalistic Realism, Rational Humanism, and positions within Catholic educational philosophy)

## II.  Ethics (Axiology)

    a.  Traditional (including elements of Strongly Traditional; Philosophic Realism, plus theology)
    b.  Progressive (Pragmatic Naturalism; Ethical Naturalism)
    c.  Analytic (Emotive Theory; "Good Reasons" Approach)
    d.  Existentialistic (atheistic, agnostic, and some Christians)
    e.  Traditional (Philosophic Idealism; Protestant Christian)
    f.  Somewhat Progressive (Brameld; Ethical Naturalism)

## III. Educational Aims and Objectives

    a.  Existentialistic
    b.  Somewhat Progressive
    c.  Analytic
    d.  Progressive
    e.  Traditional (including elements of Strongly Traditional)
    f.  Traditional

## IV.  The Educative Process (Epistemology)

    a.  Traditional
    b.  Existentialistic
    c.  Progressive
    d.  Analytic
    e.  Somewhat Progressive
    f.  Traditional (including elements of Strongly Traditional)

## V.  Physical Activity Education (including Sport)

    a.  Somewhat Progressive
    b.  Existentialistic

c. Traditional (including elements of Strongly Traditional)
d. Progressive
e. Analytic
f. Traditional

## Table 1

## Summarizing Tally Form

—  —  —  —  —  —

| Category | I | | Metaphysics |
|---|---|---|---|
| Category | II | | Ethics & Morality |
| Category | III | | Educational Objectives |
| Category | IV | | Epistemology |
| Category | V | | Physical Activity Education |

Totals    —  —  —  —  —  —

Further Instructions: It should now be possible--keeping in mind the subjectivity of an instrument such as this--to determine your position approximately based on the answers that you have given and then tallied on the form immediately above.

At the very least you should be able to tell if you are progressive, traditional, existentialistic, or analytic in your philosophic approach.

If you discover considerable eclecticism in your overall position or stance--that is, checks that place you on opposite sides of the Freedom-Constraint Spectrum, or some vacillation with checks in the existentialistic or analytic categories--you may wish then to analyze your positions or stances more closely to see if your overall position is philosophically defensible.

Keep in mind that your choices under Category I (Metaphysics or Nature of Reality) and Category II (Axiology/Values) are basic and in all probability have a strong influence on your subsequent selections.

Now please examine the Freedom-Constraint Spectrum at the beginning of this section again. Keep in mind that "Existentialistic" is not considered a position or stance as the others are (e.g., Traditional or Philosophic Idealism). Also, if you tend to be "Analytic," this means that your pre-occupation is with analysis as opposed to any "philosophical/theological" system-building.

Finally, then, after tallying the answers (your "score" above), and keeping in mind that the goal is not to "pigeonhole you forever more," did this self-evaluation checklist show you to be:

( ) Strongly Progressive--4 to 5 checks left of center on the Spectrum?

( ) Progressive--3 to 4 checks left of center?

( ) Somewhat Progressive--3 checks left of center?

( ) Eclectic--checks in 2 or 3 positions on both right and left of the Spectrum's center?

( ) Somewhat Traditional--3 checks right of center?

( ) Traditional--3 to 4 checks right of center?

( ) Strongly Traditional--4 to 5 checks right of center?

( ) Existentialistic--4 to 5 checks (including Category I) relating to this stance?

( ) Analytic--4 to 5 checks (including Category I) relating to this approach to doing

238

# Appendix B
## A Values Questionnaire for North Americans:
## Where Are You On a Socio-Political Spectrum?

## Instructions:

What really is *your* socio-political stance or position? This questionnaire will help you figure out where you really stand--not where you may nominally think that you are. When someone asks, "Are you a conservative or a liberal (or progressive)? What do you say in response? How can you justify such an answer?

> (Note: Keep in mind that these responses do not necessarily equate with the presently stated platforms of existing political parties in either the United States or Canada.)

Very few people will admit that they are radical or reactionary (i.e., far left or far right). Even if you are neutral, or middle-of-the-road, it should be possible to make that determination. Why is this important? Simply because those with an "ordered mind" ought to be able to state their beliefs and opinions with reasonable consistency throughout based on a set of comprehensible values.

Answer the following questions to the best of your ability in accordance with your reason and/or conscience. You are designating *how you want it to be!* Where possible, a position has been carefully worded to represent one of the following six positions: (1) **Reactionary**, (2) **Conservative,** (3) **Moderate Conservative**, (4) **Moderate Liberal**, (5) **Liberal**, AND (6) **Radical**. In some instances, allowing only two options for response (i.e., agreement or disagreement) was deemed best.

Please encircle the letter (a, b, etc.) that appears before the answer you select. On any given issue, a middle-of-the-road position to the right or left on a spectrum would fluctuate between +3 and +1 or between -3 and -1. When you are finished with the self-evaluation, and the scores are totaled, it should be possible for you to designate yourself one way or the other. However, you may be an *eclectic* (i.e., a person with widely distributed responses from both sides of the spectrum). Perhaps you will be a truly *middle-of-the-road person* (i.e., generally neutral on most questions).

The scoring system is included at the end of the questionnaire. In each question, please select the answer that comes the closest to reflecting ***how you would like it to be*** (!)

# Figure 1

## Where Do You Fall on the Socio-Political Spectrum?

Eclecticism*
(Maverick*)
(-6 to +6**)

| Moderate Liberal (-7 to -19) | Moderate Conservative (+7 to +19) |

Liberal (-20 to -32)                    Conservative (+20 to +32)

Radical (-33 to -45)                              Reactionary (+33 to +45)

"the left"                                              "the right"

* The so-called eclectic or "maverick" approach is placed in the center because it assumes that the person evaluating himself or herself has selected several positions on *opposite* sides of the spectrum. Most would argue that eclecticism--or a position that might be called "maverick"--is philosophically indefensible. Because of the subjectivity involved, some believe that "patterned eclecticism" (or "reasoned incoherence") represents a stance which most of us hold.

** The numerals refer to scores made on the spectrum scale.

## Question #1: THE UNITED NATIONS.

The place of the United Nations in world government should be:

a. **Negligible**--(i.e., advisory only or possibly eliminated).

b. **Minor**--and used for voluntary arbitration of international disputes only.

c. **As at present**--with members of Council having veto power.

d. **Enlarged somewhat** --and characterized by more adequate enforcement of decisions.

e. **Expanded somewhat**--and involved with actual enforcement of peacekeeping.

f. **Expanded greatly--**and hold the leading position in world government (a similar relationship as a federal government does to its states or provinces.

## Question #2: FOREIGN AID.

North Americans should:

a. Stop all foreign aid except when serious natural disasters occur.

b. Help friendly nations and/or neutral nations strengthen themselves against communistic and similar undemocratic nations by providing economic and educational assistance.

c. Provide aid to developing nations to the best of our ability, but only to those who ask for such aid and are willing to use it for sound economic development. The channeling of aid through an international agency is basic.

d. Keep foreign aid to a minimum, getting involved only when it is clearly in our self-interest.

e. Provide assistance to free and/or neutral nations only.

f. Aid economically any needy country that requests such help for basic services.

## Question #3: WAR AND PEACE.

As to military affairs and defense, North Americans should:

    a.  Work to outlaw war through unilateral disarmament by ***all*** nations.

    b.  Intervene militarily only when required (by United Nations and NATO) when the need is extreme--and then only in an effort to bring peace and to protect further loss of life.  Major powers should disarm to an "irreducible minimum."

    c.  Give military assistance to free or neutral nations when they request it. Encourage the idea of disarmament.

    d.  Help friendly and/or neutral nations with military assistance against infiltration by undemocratic ideologies (e.g., communism).

    e.  Stand prepared to protect the free world and "third– world" nations with military forces at all times.

    f.  Deal ruthlessly with naked aggression wherever it occurs (including use of nuclear power).

## Question #4: HOSTAGE CRISES.

In a hostage crisis where one country holds North American citizens at ransom (or for whatever purpose) warrants the following action:

    a.  An urgent request for an explanation, assurance of safe release, and reparation for damages at the first possible moment.

    b.  Armed invasion as soon as it becomes apparent that the hostages taken are in danger and will not be released.

    c.  A protest through diplomatic channels for an explanation with a plea for swift action and the safety of the hostages.

    d.  An immediate warning that such kidnapping and terrorist activity will not be tolerated. The foreign government concerned should understand that some direct action will be taken if hostages are not released by a specified date.

    e.  The immediate establishment of a naval blockade to the extent possible along with the implementation of other sanctions possible (e.g., freezing of assets).

    f.  A sharp protest through diplomatic channels indicating that consideration will be given to what measures might be taken to effect the release of the hostages.

## Question #5: PROTESTS AND RIOTING.

Youth, both at home and abroad, are causing considerable concern to governmental officials at all levels. I feel that young people:

    a.  Must be made to respect law and order. Rioters who loot should be warned and then shot if they do not stop. Foreign nationals, immigrants, and other marginal persons in these groups should be rooted out, jailed, and/or deported.

    b.  Are in many cases, attempting to move positively toward an improved national and international order. They should be given many different types of roles to play, as well as opportunities to improve the situation through involvement.

    c.  Are concerned and need positive leadership from adults who have experience and expertise in such matters. Only a small percent of these activists are radical and need truly firm control.

    d.  Are justified in their struggle to change the basic nature of the society. Ethnic minority groups, Blacks (in the States), and young people should not have to wait forever for much-   needed change. Many fundamental institutions must be rebuilt from the ground up.

    e.  Are proving in many cases to be ungrateful brats. Lax, frightened adults have allowed them to get out of hand too often. Strong adult leadership is required.

    f.  Are troubled and need guidance from qualified personnel. Only a relatively few are real troublemakers who need to be curbed by force. The large majority of youth will turn out to be decent, law-abiding adults.

## Question #6: PUBLIC WELFARE.

Public welfare programs in North America are:

a.  Urgently needed and should be coordinated by the federal government. There should be a guaranteed annual income for all needy families sufficient to provide a reasonable standard of living pro-rated to the cost-of-living in the geographical region involved.  Billions are needed as soon as possible to upgrade all aspects of the lives of the poor and neglected members of society.

b.  Best left to states and local governments to provide only the most needy with some assistance. Heads of families (or close relatives) should work to provide for the welfare of their families (and/or close relatives). Government handouts should be kept to an absolute minimum.

c.  Needed on a limited basis from all levels of government, but experience has shown that the federal government should set and enforce national standards. In this way, all families will have sufficient resources to maintain at least a minimum standard of living. Current disincentives to work must somehow be removed.

d.  Unfortunately necessary. Somehow the current disincentives toward work must be eliminated. All male and female recipients should be worked back into the job force--even by doing public service work for their welfare payments. Perhaps by introducing national or regional standards that take into consideration cost of living indexes in the various "high" welfare states.

e. Positively dangerous to the future of our democratic societies on the continent because they are inexorably bringing about a decay of moral fiber. In our North American culture people work for a living. We must become firmer. If those currently on the dole get hungry enough, they will find some work to do to support themselves and their families.

f.  A "sop" to mislead the poor and trick them into acceptance of the capitalist system. The nation's wealth should be redistributed so as to assure virtual equality for all people who are willing to be gainfully employed citizens. The current systematic degradation and exploitation of the poor must stop.

## Question #7: FREEDOM OF SPEECH AND PRESS.

The rights of freedom of speech and press contained, for example, in the First Amendment of the U.S. Constitution:

a. Are part of the heritage of free men and women on this continent, but subversive and immoral elements have been allowed to take advantage of these rights. Certain people and related social influences threaten to destroy the fabric of freedom.

b. Are a vital part of the America's and Canada's heritage. We all profit from new and different ideas. However, it is necessary to limit speech and action that present a "clear and present danger" to our civil and moral welfare.

c. Are perhaps the most important rights granted to citizens by government in constitutions and bills of right. Movements to dilute or "balance away" these rights in the interest of national security have typically been misdirected. Suppression of speech and movement should be carried out only in extreme situations.

d. Are a part of the democratic heritage in the United States, but freedom does not mean license to say anything one wants to say at any time. There must be strong checks on pornography or revolutionary speech and action.

e. Are a myth because the corporate, capitalistic power structure through employment of the mass media conspires to suppress free and creative speech and thought.

f. Were grossly misinterpreted by past Supreme Court judgments. All obscene and subversive materials and actions must be suppressed to protect our country from the radical revolutionary threat at home and the planned world take-over elsewhere.

## Question #8: ECONOMICS & BUSINESS.

Please read the following statement carefully. Then try to categorize yourself in one of the ways indicated.

One of the first concerns of a federal government in North America should be the provision of a sound business climate. This is accomplished best if the government employs only minimum restrictions on businesses and corporations

For example, wage and hour legislation is wrong. Any contract that developed—if there must be one—should be arranged strictly between employers and employees.

Concurrently, every effort should be made to stay with a balanced budget. In fact, an economy will not really be (safe and) sound until steady, sensible fiscal policies bring about a significant reduction in a national debt. However, it is important, also, not to increase the burden on taxpayers even though a strong national defense is necessary. Big business is taxed so heavily that people's dividends on their investments are becoming unreasonably small. Inflation must stay at a reasonable level, and the economy needs ever-present stimulation.

Through reasonable policies about spending both at home and abroad, we should be able to develop a type of revenue—sharing in the years ahead. Through the stimulation of private enterprise, with occasional block grants of money with no strings attached made to states or provinces ha are hard pressed financially, we should be able to improve the economy with a *minimum* of revenue-sharing that is ultimately debilitating to struggling state/provincial and local political units. We must strive always to keep people's money closer to the source from which produces it in the first place. A federal government simply cannot be "all things to all people." It is time that many of the required responsibilities and duties be returned to the state/province along with the necessary tax money to carry these tasks forward to successful conclusion,

a. **I agree** with just about all of the ideas of the ideas expressed in this statement.

b. **I disagree generally** with this statement, To me the tone seems negative. I feel that the federal government should become more involved in the control of business and industry.

c, **I disagree** with the statement. *Laissez faire* capitalism certainly helped this country initially to become strong materially. Now, however, we need somewhat more of a social-welfare state approach to meet the urgent needs of a significant percentage of the people.

d. **I agree generally** with this statement. It seems quite sensible and reasonable. It offers positive recommendations to alleviate some of the ongoing problems that we face.

e. **I disagree strongly**. Much of this statement is reactionary drivel. Some of these ideas may have made some sense back in the 19th century. However, the super-rich and the rich have "gotten away with murder" in North America. We simply have to figure out a way to redistribute the wealth to a reasonable extent. Democratic socialism is the answer.

f. **I agree strongly.** The labor movement and extended welfare programs have had a lot to do with the sad fiscal plight of both the United States and Canada. Budgets should be balanced, but they never will be with so many inadequate, lazy people living off the fat of the land on, for example, huge governmental payrolls. People simply must prepare themselves *and be willing* to work. Maybe being hungry will make them look a little harder for any gainful employment.

## Question #9: LAW AND ORDER.

Law and order is:

a. **Necessary to maintain an organized healthy society**. The lack of respect for authority has led to many unfortunate incidents at all levels of society. The Supreme Court in the United States, for example, went too far in interpreting the constitutional rights of criminals. Canada has done the same. Maybe now we'll gradually firm up our defenses against the rising tide of people who have no fear of inadequate punishments that will be meted out to them.

b. **The emotional slogan of many of those individuals and groups who oppose progressive social change**. Law and order without justice is characteristic of totalitarian societies. There should be no wire tapping at all, for example. Although rioting can't be condoned, it is essential that we attack the causes of such insurrection--not the symptoms of unrest that might be inherent in present society.

c. **Essential if the free countries of the world are to survive this very difficult period**. For a variety of reasons, legislatures and "supreme courts" have gone too far in coddling the truly dangerous criminal offenders without regard to public safety. In some instances, jurisdictions have even gone so far as to pay criminals to reveal where they have hidden bodies of their victims.

d. **The hypocritical slogan of a frightened and decadent society**. The poor and minority groups occasionally strike back at the absolute, but often

concealed, viciousness of an exploitive social order. "Law-'n order" tends to mean "keep
Black, multi-ethnic minorities, youth, and immigrants in their place!" We must treat all alike in our society.

e. **The backbone of a free society**. Absolutely no gains should be allowed as a result of rioting and looting with protests that get out of hand. Civil disturbances must be suppressed ruthlessly. Too many "handcuffs" have been placed on members of law-enforcement agencies doing their jobs. Maybe once again women will all be able to walk the streets without fear of molestation.

f. **Necessary in a democratic society, but the words as used by many take on an unpleasant overtone**. Crimes rates of several types are really serious, but we must move positively rather than negatively to reach their causes and then correct them. Prison rehabilitation programs must be improved significantly. I believe that crime rates would go down markedly if competency-based education and more jobs were made available.

## Question #10  POPULATION CONTROL.
Please read the following paragraph. Then indicate the strength or your agreement or disagreement with the import of the statement.

The population control is starkly grim today. The situation has become now become so tragic because there are more than six billion people on earth--and the projection figure is nine billion before a declining trend is expected. We are told that all-out cooperative efforts by the major powers in the world simply cannot ward off the massive starvation of peoples that is coming in the years ahead.

Even if nutrition of an adequate nature were somehow to be provided, over-population is also causing staggering problems with water and stream pollution, air pollution, overcrowding in cities, etc. These difficulties will steadily great worse. A crisis of this magnitude must obviously be attacked on all fronts by people of good will worldwide.

The right to abortion should be legalized universally and readily available when there is no desire to carry a fetus through to birth. The sole choice in this matter should rest with the prospective parents (the mother in the final analysis) with advice from a physician when requested.

Coeducational sex education should be carried out in the public schools at the earliest appropriate age. Contraceptive advice , devices when requested, should be readily available and kept at an inexpensive level with governmental subsidy if required. Subsequently, in overpopulated countries, it will probably be necessary to offer positive incentives--or even penalties!--so that the size of families will be curtailed.

Finally, we can't make the point too strongly that this vital matter has a direct relationship to world peace. There is absolutely no time to waste in the implementation of the necessary procedures to carry out the underlying philosophy expressed in the above statements.

a. **Agreement**--The underlying rationality of this statement and the specific steps to be taken represent my position. Action is needed as soon as possible.

b. **Disagreement**--This is a highly personal matter. The government should refrain from direct involvement. The problem may be serious in a relatively small number of countries, but they should be able to solve it with intelligent planning.

c. **Strong Agreement**--This position and the implementation of the accompanying recommendations represent just a beginning. All sorts of additional measures will be needed in the future. For example, why shouldn't we have licensing so that only genetically qualified people will be allowed to bring children into the world?

d. **Strong Disagreement**--this statement is ridiculous! It goes on at length about something that really isn't a problem. If God had meant for people to be controlled as to the number of offspring they may produce, it would have been so. Government has absolutely no right to become involved in such an aspect of a woman's life (or that of her mate). This whole trend should be resisted very strongly.

e. **Agree Generally**--population control is certainly one of the world's problems. We should work to improve the situation at home and encourage other nations to do the same.

f. **Disagree Generally**--Many have expressed concern about this problem, but it really is not as serious as they have indicated. Birth control information should be available on a voluntary basis to those whose religious faith permits such a practice.

## Question #11  TRADE UNIONS.

Identify the extent of your agreement or disagreement with the following statement:

The origin, growth, and development of trade unions in North America have been most significant. When the capitalistic system reached a stage where large individual fortunes were being made, certain segments of the working population were finding it next to impossible to realize the material benefits necessary to maintain a reasonable and secure standard of living.

The advances made by unions did not come easily. In fact, the struggle was exceedingly difficult. Often long, bitter strikes were needed before reasonable--not always equitable--settlements were effected. These periodic strikes brought great hardships to many families. The concept of a "closed shop" was a bitter pill for many companies and industries to swallow. It still is for many today. The establishment of a relationship between salary raises and the cost-of-living index did not come easily either. Most helpful to the development of unions was their informal yet strong tie-ins with political parties.

The union movement has spread in many directions. This development has been very helpful to such groups as government workers, teachers, and many other occupations. Union leaders and rank-and-file members should now make strong efforts to recruit members of minority groups, women, and any other needy people at all levels of the business and commercial enterprise. This must be done, even if it becomes necessary to change existing standards temporarily--or perhaps brought about by setting up a larger number of categories. If a capitalistic economy is to exist worldwide, unions must loom large in the struggle for equality of opportunity here and everywhere else.

Unions should continue with the vigorous prosecution of their demands for such benefits as the guaranteed annual wage and other rewards to enable workers to steadily improve their quality of life. The government should not invoke the idea of compulsory arbitration except in most extreme situations to settle longstanding disputes, nor should it subject unions to back-to-work legislation except when a national emergency exists.

a.  **Agreement**--This is my position. The union movement gives me hope that the world is a fair place in which to live. Unions have given workers a sense of security and morale that permits them to work more productively and comfortably at the same time.

b.  **General Disagreement**--There are some good points here, but this statement gives unions far too much credit and power.

c.  **Strong Disagreement**--This is ridiculous. The power of the unions must be curbed before the overall economy is destroyed.

d.  **General Agreement**--The unions have helped North American companies, but some of these statements go too far. No group should be allowed to become too powerful.

e.  **Disagreement**--This is definitely not my belief about the background and present position of trade unions. Union development needs to be watched carefully for excesses that are apt to creep in.

f.  **Strong Agreement**--This statement is good, but the report of accomplishments should be even more glowing. The United States and Canada would not be where they are today if it were not for the magnificent saga of North America's trade unions.

## Question #12  HIGHLY COMPETITIVE SPORT.

Please record the extent to which you agree or  disagree with the following statement:

Competitive sport was created by people thousands of years ago (presumably) to serve humankind beneficially. It can and does serve a multitude of purposes in today's world.  With sound leadership it can good for both boys and girls in their formative years. It can help to develop desirable character and personality traits and also promote vigorous health. It can also provide good role models for young people to emulate. Our states and provinces should get fully behind these activities by providing appropriate competition for young people as they are developing. Such sporting competition should be regarded as supplemental to regular physical activity education programs at all levels of education.

To compete in highly competitive sport today, and do well, it requires extensive, dedicated practice over a period of many years. It is argued that it is important for our countries to be well represented in international competitions and at the Olympic Games. Thus, we should continue to find ways that we can more fully subsidize our young people so that they may strive for, and perhaps ultimately achieve their highest aspirations in this regard. Eventually a small percentage of these athletes will, in addition to the *intrinsic* rewards that sport participation provides, will search for ways to capitalize *extrinsically*, also on any such talent developed. In certain sports particularly enjoyed by society, these young people may even turn professional as such status becomes available to them.

Such a development takes place in a number of other life activities (e.g., music, drama), but in sport in the past, this was somehow contrary to the amateur ideal and the spirit of Olympism. However, holding true to the original Olympic ideal has just about become impossibility today. When the United States, for example, lost the Olympic title in basketball, there evidently could be only one response--bring in the "pros" with their multi-million salaries to trounce those "upstarts." Now even they are having trouble "bringing home the bacon!"

As the Olympic Movement becomes increasingly professionalized at all levels, along with the problem of controlling drug usage to enhance performance, one wonders to what extent present-day practices can be compared to the problems that arose with the ancient Olympic Games. They were abolished in 776 B.C. because of the excesses that developed. We must search harder for ways to hold this cheating and phony "professionalism" in check? The question arises: Will the modern Games suffer the same fate as those in ancient times for similar reasons?

a. **Agreement--**This is a very good statement. Sport can indeed be a force for *good* in the world, but we must be very careful to ensure that the *evil present* in many of the prevailing practices that have developed with highly commercialized sport doesn't outweigh any good that might be achieved. We are dangerously close to this now wherever the emphasis is on money largely and not on what is happening to the young man or woman involved. Many of these influences have "trickled down" to certain universities and some schools at the lower levels. We need fine programs of intramural sports for young people in all school.

b. **Disagreement--**This statement has some merit, but I do not buy this "good and evil" bit as described immediately above. Competitive sport has proved itself an important social influence in society. It is important to have as many "winners" as possible in today's world. It is a "hard" world out there, and people need to know how to compete. In addition, it is vital for our country to do well in international competition including the involvement with the Olympic Games. Further, young people who can earn athletic scholarships for their university education deserve this chance. Additionally, highly competitive sport provides a great deal of entertainment and enjoyment to millions of people as well.

**Question #13--GAY AND LESBIAN RELATIONSHIPS**. Please read the following statement carefully, and then decide which position or stance is closest to your present values and beliefs.

Morality and ethics have been hot topics from the 1990s on into the new century. *The New York Times* reported, for example, "our morality is disintegrating because its foundation is eroding." The Washington Post asserted, "The core of U.S. national character has been damaged because we've lost our sense of virtue!" Although denying a person's right to choose abortion is still being argued by a minority, the question of gays in the military has been only temporarily (quite unsatisfactorily) resolved in the U.S.A. In addition, we are still finding difficulty in granting full rights as citizens to same-sex alliances. Of course, it does seem reasonable that, if a person is willing to die for his or her country in military service, how this person fulfills sexual desires in the privacy of a bedroom should hardly be a major issue today. Nevertheless, the questions of immorality and its relationship to the legal system are still present and will not go away easily.

John Kekes, a U.S. philosopher, calls the argument that "the world is going to Hell in a hand basket," morally speaking, The *Disintegration Thesis*. The position is as follows:

(1) The value system of the culture no longer offers significant rationale for subordinating one's self to the common good.
(2) A healthy democratic government depends on values that come from religion (the Judeo-Christian tradition that is).
(3) Human rights are based on the moral worth that a loving God has granted to each human soul.
(4) Authority in social affairs is empowered because of underlying transcendent moral law (Brookings Institution).

What this all adds up to is that the Disintegration Thesis holds since society's basic problem is moral. What rebuttal may be offered to the idea that our culture is sliding down a slippery slope to moral bankruptcy? Kekes argues that the whole problem is simply this: Moral change has been confused with moral disintegration. He agrees that are many seemingly disturbing moral issues today, but he then inquires about the significance of these facts as a "new morality" struggles to be born. What is being abandoned is the idea that there is one and only one set of virtues for a human life--One *Summum Bonum*, to place the dilemma in terms of Latin.

However, the Disintegration Thesis argument is that a gradual change in our morality has been occurring, and that such change will continue into the future. However, in this change from a single morality to a pluralistic one in North America, there are still many good traits or virtues present in our daily lives. We still have the basic concepts of freedom, knowledge, happiness, justice, love, order, privacy, wisdom, etc. with which to guide and develop our personal lives and social living. However, we should understand that in this ever-increasing pluralistic culture none of these concepts is necessarily reducible to the other--and especially not to the idea that there is one transcendental moral law. This means that each person should work in his or her life for some reasonable or acceptable combination of such values as love, freedom, justice, etc.

a. **Agreement**. I find myself essentially in agreement with the position taken immediately above by the writer. Times are indeed changing, and we simply must be fair to *all* concerned. A number of the concerns expressed about gay and lesbian relationships are not central to "the good life"--they are peripheral. What is important in life is that we should be fair, decent, and just in our relationships with others--not that we should concern ourselves with people's sexual preferences. A spectrum seems to exist about the "maleness" or "femaleness" of a person, a condition that is inherent in that individual and cannot be altered without maladjustment occurring.

b. **Disagreement.** This "NEW" morality sounds great and may be fine to those individuals ready to accept the changes that are occurring toward a pluralistic morality. However, as a defender of The Disintegration Thesis, this argument for acceptance of such an oddly emerging situation simply adds fuel to the fire. Any individually selected amalgam of values and virtues represents just one more symptom of the moral bankruptcy that is taking place right before our eyes. The advocates of a new, more pluralistic morality, if they hope to win their argument, must show that there is sufficient continuity between the old and the new, between monistic and pluralistic morality.

## Question #14 ENVIRONMENTAL CRISIS.

Please read the following statement. Then decide which of the two statements below is closest to your stance or belief about the problem outlined.

Ecology is defined as the field of study that treats the relationships and interactions of human beings and other living organisms with each other and with their natural environment. Since 1975, interest in this vital subject has increased steadily and markedly with each passing year. Nevertheless, the "say-do" gap in relation to truly doing something about Earth's plight in this regard is enormous.

What, then, is the extent of the environmental crisis in modern society? Very simply, we have achieved a certain mastery over the world because of our scientific and technological achievement. We are at the top of the food chain because of our mastery of much of Earth's flora and fauna. However, because of the explosion of the human population, increasingly greater pressures "will be placed on our lands to provide shelter, food, recreation, and waste disposal areas. This will cause a greater pollution of the atmosphere, the rivers, the lakes, the land, and the oceans" (Mergen). This bleak picture could be expanded; yet, perhaps the tide will soon turn. Certainly many recognize the gravity of prevailing patterns of human conduct, but a great many more people must develop attitudes that will lead them to take positive action in the immediate future. It is time for concerted global action, and we can only hope that it is not too late to reverse the effects of a most grave situation.

We can all appreciate the difficulty of moving from a scientific "is" to an ethical "ought" in the realm of human affairs. There are obviously many scientific findings within the environmental sciences that should be made available to people of all ages. Simply making the facts available, of course, will not be any guarantee that strong and positive attitudes will develop on the subject. It is a well-established fact, however, that the passing of legislation in difficult and sensitive areas must take place through responsible political leadership, and that attitude changes often follow behind, albeit at what may seem to be a snail's pace.

The field of education should play a vital role now, as it has never done before, in the development of what might be called an "ecological awareness." Obviously, this has become much broader than it was earlier because the field of ecology now places all of the individual entities of Earth in a total context in which the interrelationship of all parts must be thoroughly understood. If the field of education has a strong obligation to present the various issues revolving about the newly understood need for the development of an ecological awareness, this duty obviously includes all who are employed within the educational system, have a certain general education responsibility to all participants in their classes or programs.

Presumably, this matter cannot be called a persistent problem historically. The overwhelming magnitude of poor ecological practices has not been even partially understood by the general populace. Now some realize the urgency of the matter, but others are telling them that further study is needed, that the ecologists are exaggerating, and that they are simply pessimistic by nature.

a. **Agreement.** I find myself in essential agreement with the underlying position taken by the writer above. This is a crisis because the need for "ecological awareness" is racing headlong into a collision with growing worldwide capitalism in the burgeoning global economy. The time is now to take drastic steps to alleviate and/or resolve this overwhelmingly difficult problem.

b. **Disagreement**. The writer makes some good points, of course. We must be ever vigilant as to elements and forces (also companies and people) that are careless and/or dishonest in their "relations" with the environment. However, if a country seeks to do conscientiously what it can to alleviate problems that develop, that should do the trick. The earth is resilient. This is one of a number of important and issues the world is facing.

**Question #15 CLONING AND CELLULAR RESEARCH.** Please read the statement below. Then record your agreement or disagreement as you did with previous questions.

In the 21st century, using a Biblical-quoting rationale based on Genesis (IV), to castigate scientists for "staggering arrogance" in presuming to play God by conducting cloning research does not cut much ice. (Note that god is spelled with a capital "G.") As the argument proceeds, none other than the eminent philosopher/theologian, George W. Bush, bolsters the strength of this argument. Does the author actually think that this former Yale "scholar" personally wrote-- and indeed meant! --the words he spoke? "As we seek what is possible, we must also ask what is right--and we must not forget that even the most noble ends do not justify any means".

In response, here is a thought for our nay saying friends to absorb early in this new millennium. Your Christian God has a tough struggle ahead to keep its status as the number #1 life force in a multiethnic world. The world society is just too replete with its many versions of "The Great One." This is becoming ever more true as both Europeans and North Americans struggle with their own rapidly increasing, multiethnic cultural incursions. Each has its "unique" version of the Almighty.

When it comes to this question of cellular and cloning research, the voices of the clerics involved come through as a "vast pooling of ignorance." They speak as though they KNOW what is right and what is wrong. They know, you see, because God told them so! The fact of the matter is that neither they--nor do any of the rest of us as their often gullible listeners--really know what is right and what is wrong anymore. Their hoary dogma simply does not "do it" today.

Unless knowledge of "how it all began" somehow becomes known to humankind–and can we really believe this will ever happen? --we earthlings do not have much choice. We must figure out--working together! --what's "right" action and what's "wrong" action for us in the 21st century. Our decisions quite simply must be **based on our own life experience**. If we do not manage to do this, ultimate disaster to life as we know it today seems almost inevitable. The handwriting is on the wall!

Cross-cultural understanding must be cultivated with great diligence. This is vital because our "global village" with its blanketing communications network is steadily bringing about similar values and norms of conduct worldwide. The world needs to view solutions to ethical dilemmas such as cloning and cellular research in a similar manner. Such an approach to ethical decision-making could well be the only hope for human life to continue successfully on Earth in the future.

a. **Agreement**. Findings from the scientific community keep flooding in. Some are good, some debatable, and some turn out to be wrong. Life moves on in often strange and mysterious ways. It appears to be an open-ended universe. We do not really know where we came from, or where we are going. Scientific discoveries and the medical profession backed by the health sciences have lengthened the average length of human life. Now we are promised even better length and longevity through cellular research. I say, "Go for it!"

b. **Disagreement**. How far should humans go in tampering with life processes? When a man and woman are married and subsequently procreate, they are in tune with the plan that the Creator has preordained for humans and all other living creatures on earth. Humans should not tamper with His plan for us. Abortion, for example, is a sin against humankind. Using cloned creatures for "spare parts" when or where needed is not my idea of how humans should behave.

## Question #16. UNIVERSAL HEALTH CARE
Please read the statement below. Then record your agreement or disagreement as you did with previous questions.

So-called "universal health care" is now a great problem for countries of the world to solve. This is so because the expense of paying for all sorts of medical expenses, including some based on incomplete scientific backing, has become prohibitive. To pay for everything "eats up" a "disproportionate" amount of as country's overall budget.

In North America, for example, the United States has a situation in which some 45% of the population has no medical coverage. In addition, it is not known what percentage of the remainder have policies that provide that could be termed "inadequate" coverage. Often when a specific claim is made, the response is that either coverage is not available on the existing policy, or that only a percentage of the needed amount will be paid.

The Canadian situation is different in that all bona fide residents have universal health care. However, provision of such "universality" is now a problem of increasing concern because of the enormous expense involved. Fortunately, all life-threatening illnesses are cared for as "emergencies" at the first possible moment. However, it is "elective" surgery and other "non-emergency" care that have become a problem because of long waiting periods for treatment. In addition, each province has different arrangements as to which "unproven," but possibly helpful service or medication will be covered under the medical insurance plan.

A further issue has arisen as well. Private agencies are developing plans whereby people with the necessary means can get treatment for so-called "elective" medical problems much sooner that if they simply waited their turn. A variation of this view of the issue is a scheme whereby a person can get insurance to cover his/her expense (and that of a companion) to travel to the United States for treatment IF service is not available in Canada after a specified period.

Everything considered, in the 21st country a North American country ought to provide full medical coverage for all of its citizens regardless of their ability to pay. Not to do so creates a situation in which the needs of rich people are met in one way or another, The needs of the middle-class may be met, but some times by incurring long term-debt. In addition, the poor simply "fade away" and die sooner. The only fair and just conclusion is that the total expense should be borne by the government through its taxation scheme.

a. **Agreement.** I believe that medical coverage should be "complete" for *all* to the greatest possible extent. The time has past when a modern country should have "first-class" citizens and "second-class" citizens when it comes to a person's health and wellbeing.

b. **Disagreement**. I certainly do not want to see people suffer unnecessarily or die because of inadequate medical care. However, government simply cannot be "all things to all people at all times." People have to learn to become responsible citizens. They need to plan their budgets carefully so that they and their families will be provided for in the various circumstances that arise. Emergency coverage is one thing that the government should be responsible for, but complete insurance coverage for all sorts of elective medical services is more than a person has a right to expect in our society.

## Question #17. EDUCATIONAL AIMS & OBJECTIVES
The fundamental aim of education is:

a. Education should seek to "awaken awareness" in the learner (i.e., awareness of the person as a single subjectivity in the world. Increased emphasis is needed on the arts and social sciences, and the student should freely and creatively choose his or her own pattern of education. Socialization of the child has become equally as important as his or her intellectual development as a key educational aim in this century.

b. Social-self-realization is the supreme value in education. The realization of this ideal is most important for the individual in the social setting--a world culture. Positive ideals should be molded toward the evolving democratic ideal by a general education that is group-centered and in which the majority determines the acceptable goals. However, once that majority opinion is determined, all are obligated to conform until such majority opinion can be reversed (the doctrine of "defensible partiality").

c. The concept of 'education' has become much more complex that was ever realized before. Because of the various meanings of the term "education," talking about educational aims and objectives is almost a hopeless task unless a myriad of qualifications is used for clarification. We need to qualify our meaning to explain to the listener whether we mean (1) the subject-matter; (2) the activity of education carried on by teachers; (3) the process of being educated (or learning) that is occurring; (4) the result, actual or intended, or No.2 and No.3 Immediately above taking place through the employment of that which comprises No.1 above; (5) the discipline, or field of enquiry and investigation; and (6) the profession whose members are involved professionally with all of the aspects of education described above. With this understanding, it is then possible to make some determination about which specific objectives the profession of education should strive for as it moves in the direction of the achievement of long range aims.

d. The general aim of education is more education. Education in the broadest sense can be nothing else than the changes made in human beings by their experience. Participation by students in the formation of aims and objectives is essential to generate the all-important desired interest required for the finest educational process to occur. Social efficiency (i.e., societal socialization) should be considered the general aim of education. Pupil growth is a paramount goal. This means that the individual is placed at the center of the educational experience.

e. The aim of education is the acquisition of verified knowledge of the individual's environment. This aim recognizes the value of content as well as the activities involved; and also takes into account the external determinants of human behavior. Education is the acquisition of the art of the utilization of knowledge. The primary task of education is to transmit knowledge, knowledge without which civilization could not continue to flourish. Some holding this philosophy believe that the good life emanates from cooperation with God's grace, and believe further that the development of these virtues is obviously of greater worth than learning or anything else.

f. Through education the developing organism becomes what it latently is. All education has a religious significance, the meaning of which is that there is a "moral imperative" on education. As the person's mind strives to realize itself, there is the possibility of the Absolute within the individual mind. Education should aid the child to adjust to the basic realities (the spiritual ideals of truth, beauty, and goodness) that the history of the race has furnished us. The basic values of human living are health, character, social justice, skill, art, love, knowledge, philosophy, and religion.

++++++++++++++++++++++++++++++++++++++++++++++++

*See next page for scoring instructions*

**Check your answers with the following Score Sheet. With each question write in the appropriate number of points scored (*as plus or minus*) where indicated.**

| Question | | | | Question | | | |
|---|---|---|---|---|---|---|---|
| 1. | a. | +3 | | 6. | a. | -2 | |
| | b. | +2 | | | b. | +2 | |
| | c. | +1 | | | c. | -1 | |
| | d. | -1 | _____ | | d. | +1 | _____ |
| | e. | -2 | score | | e. | +3 | score |
| | f. | -3 | | | f. | -3 | |
| 2. | a. | +3 | | 7. | a. | +2 | |
| | b. | +1 | | | b. | -1 | |
| | c. | -2 | | | c. | -2 | |
| | d. | +2 | _____ | | d. | +1 | _____ |
| | e. | -1 | score | | e. | -3 | score |
| | f. | -3 | | | f. | +3 | |
| 3. | a. | -3 | | 8. | a. | +2 | |
| | b. | -2 | | | b. | -1 | |
| | c. | -1 | | | c. | -2 | |
| | d. | +1 | _____ | | d. | +1 | _____ |
| | e. | +2 | score | | e. | -3 | score |
| | f. | +3 | | | f. | +3 | |
| 4. | a. | -3 | | 9. | a. | +1 | |
| | b. | +3 | | | b. | -1 | |
| | c. | -2 | | | c. | +2 | |
| | d. | +1 | _____ | | d. | -3 | _____ |
| | e. | +2 | score | | e. | +3 | score |
| | f. | -1 | | | f. | -2 | |
| 5. | a. | +3 | | 10. | a. | -2 | |
| | b. | -2 | | | b. | +2 | |
| | c. | +1 | _____ | | c. | -3 | |
| | d. | -3 | score | | d. | -1 | _____ |
| | e. | +2 | | | e. | +1 | score |
| | f. | -1 | | | f. | +3 | |

11.  a.  -2
     b.  +1
     c.  +3
     d.  -1  _____
     e.  +2  score
     f.  -3

12.  a.  +3
     b.  -3
     c.  -2
     d.  +1  _____
     e.  -1  score
     f.  +2

13.  a.  -3
     b.  +3  _____
              score

14.  a.  -3
     b.  +3  _____
              score

15.  a.  -3
     b.  +3  _____
              score

16.  a.  -3
     b.  +3  _____
              score

17.  a.  -1 (Existentialistic)
     b.  -2 (Somewhat Progressive)
     c.  -0 (Analytic)
     d.  -3 (Progressive)
     e.  +3 (Traditional         _____
              (including Strongly Traditional Elements)   score
     f.  +2 (Traditional)

B.  Add your plus (+) scores together (if any)..........Total = _____

C.  Add your minus (-) scores together (if any).......Total = _____

D.  Subtract the smaller score (plus or minus) from the larger one.

It may be, of course, that you will have just one cumulative plus or minus score. In this case, no subtraction is necessary.

Your resultant total could conceivable be zero (0).
It is more likely, however, that it will either be plus "something" (e.g., plus [+] 9) or minus "something" (e.g., minus (-) 14.

E.  The result is your **S**ocio-**P**olitical **Q**uotient (either conservative **+ SPQ** or liberal **- SPQ**.

**Note: Of course, *this is not a good or Alternatively, bad score--whatever it is!***

***Please see the next page for a discussion of your result.***

## Discussion

Your score could range from plus 51 to minus 51. There is a world of difference between these two extremes. The scale below is a rough approximation indicating the range of socio-political "positions." Six such positions have been identified for the purposes of this self-evaluation questionnaire.

It has been argued that a country needs both socio-political conservatives **and** liberals. Progressives are anxious to see implemented what they regard as beneficial, while conservatives want to make certain that such change being recommended is desirable and possibly beneficial **before** they accept it.

A score somewhere around the zero (0) mark is difficult to assess. It probably indicates someone who is a middle-of-the-road person, perhaps a fence sitter on controversial issues. However, it might indicate someone who has varying positions on both sides of the spectrum--and whose scores simply balance each other out. This would be the position of an eclectic, but not what has been termed a patterned eclectic.

**+36 to +51**         **= (Reactionary)**

**+22 to +35**         **= (Conservative)**

**+7 to +21**         **= (Moderate Conservative)**

**+6 to -6**         **= (Middle of the Road: Eclectic or**
                                     ***Maverick?*])**

**-7 to -21**         **= (Moderate Liberal**

**-22 to -35**         **= (Liberal)**

**-36 to -51**         **= (Radical)**